aromatherapy in practice

Your introduction to the wonderful world of Aromatherapy

Ben Orr & Zoë Green

Aromatherapy in practice
Your introduction to the wonderful world of Aromatherapy

ISBN: 978-0-9928488-0-4

PUBLISHED BY
KINGSOWN PUBLISHING
Unity Street
St Phillips
Bristol
BS2 0HN
United Kingdom

Spring Equinox, 2014 CE

PRINTED AND BOUND BY CPI GROUP (UK) LTD, CROYDON CR0 4YY

ORDERING INFORMATION: Please email sales@kingsowncosmetics.com

WHOLESALES ARE AVAILABLE ON QUANTITY PURCHASES BY BOOKSHOPS, CORPORATIONS, ASSOCIATIONS AND OTHERS. PLEASE EMAIL FOR DETAILS

The authors would like to thank Rosie & James Bell
for their excellent work on the design of the book.

Also Peter Carroll for assistance and guidance.

Thanks also to Jenny Winfield, Andy Winfield,
Rory Lowings, Woody Evans, Roger Marsh,
Eugény Couture and everyone else who has
helped and advised during the creation of this book.

Finally, thanks to our respective friends and family
for emotional support and encouragement.

aromatherapy in practice

Your introduction to the wonderful world of Aromatherapy

Ben Orr & Zoë Green

about the authors

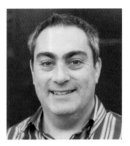

Ben Orr:
Ben has been working in the Aromatherapy business for 5 years and has long been passionate about the power and effectiveness of natural products such as essential oils. Having seen at first hand the untold benefits and positive impact that Aromatherapy can have he is constantly enthused by the opportunity to learn more about the subject and pass on his ever increasing knowledge to other people.

Aromatherapy techniques range from the incredibly simple (such as just adding a few drops to a warm bath) to some of the more complicated massage techniques. Perhaps the most positive aspect is that anyone can learn the basics relatively quickly and start providing genuinely effective treatments for themselves, family and friends.

A father to two lively, healthy boys and husband to Sue, the family regularly practises Aromatherapy at home – which is a grand way of saying they burn or vaporise essential oils nearly every day and often blend massage solutions as and when required.

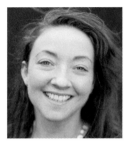

Zoë Green:
Coming from a farming family, Zoë was raised with a deep bond to the land, the seasons and nature itself. In her early years she was often found in the garden inspecting (and nibbling) flowers and foliage. This fascination has remained and Zoë has an innate ability for recognising different plant species, recalling their uses and lore.

Blessed with sensitive skin, Zoë took an interest in what cosmetics and toiletries really contain. It became clear that some ingredients did not suit her and she began to research different options for her health and well-being. Slowly yet surely she gathered lots of information, techniques and found cosmetic brands that were more in line with her needs.

By a twist of fate she gained employment at a leading UK Aromatherapy wholesaler, running their small shop. Here Zoë was able to increase her working knowledge of essential oils and carrier oils. There was a light bulb moment when she first made her own bespoke skincare products. From there, many experiments ensued (not all of them successful!). She learnt that not every oil works for every person, but there will be always a next best fit which addresses underlying reasons for conditions and the adage that less can be more.

aromatherapy in practice

Aided by practical usage, assisting clients, harnessing intuition and lots of reading Zoë has found that 'plants in bottles' really can make a profound difference to our well-being. Often sought out for advice, she feels honoured to help clients to improve their own health from simple moisturisers through to chronic condition management.

Zoë believes now, more than ever, that nature in its many wondrous forms holds the keys to unlocking our true well-being, vibrancy and happiness.

We trust that you will enjoy reading this book and that it helps you to understand some of the many ways in which you can benefit from essential oils and other natural products. We hope you are encouraged to start your own journey through the wonderful world of natural Aromatherapy.

Consultant Aromatherapist

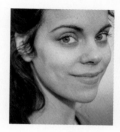

Eugény Couture: Eugény works for one of the biggest Aromatherapy companies in the UK having moved to the country from her native France 3 years ago. Her lifelong interest in Aromatherapy started at a young age in the French countryside and continued through adolescence and adulthood. On moving to England Eugény became a qualified Aromatherapist and was delighted to be asked to become involved in the creation of this book as the consultant Aromatherapist.

Eugény is happy to recommend this text as an excellent introduction to the wonderful world of Aromatherapy and is sure that it will help those who are interested in developing their own skills and abilities in using pure essential oils and other natural products to improve the health and well-being of themselves and their families.

aromatherapy in practice

aromatherapy in practice

contents

section one	an introduction to essential oils	12
	- a history	14
	- how oils are produced	22
section two	how to use essential oils	26
section three	dilution rates	34
section four	essential oils	38
section five	absolute & precious oils	106
section six	carrier oils	118
section seven	floral waters	126
section eight	physical aromatherapy	132
section nine	psychological aromatherapy	142
	disclaimer	148
	stockists	150
	glossary	154
	bibliography	158
	notes	160
	index	168

an introduction to essential oils

a history

Aromatherapy is: The use of natural ingredients, such as essential oils and herbal extracts, to create treatments which promote mental and physical well-being.

Pure essential oils are extracted by various methods from many different plants. Each oil has its own individual profile which means that there is an essential oil for pretty much every conceivable problem.

Aromatherapy is now used extensively alongside modern medicinal techniques as more and more people recognise the benefits of using the power of nature as well as the power of science.

Whereas conventional medicine practices concentrate mainly on fixing physical symptoms, Aromatherapy treatments take a more holistic view

and are aimed at easing and soothing the mental issues often associated with illness as well as the physical problems themselves.

Aromatherapy beginnings: The term Aromatherapy was only introduced around 100 years ago but it's thought that humans have been utilising the natural benefits of plants and oils since the first of our species evolved.

There is evidence that the first humans to evolve on Earth used plants as medicine and for other health benefits.

Archaeologists have discovered traces of plants that we now know have medicinal and therapeutic properties in the burial and dwelling sites of the earliest humans from around 400,000 years ago.

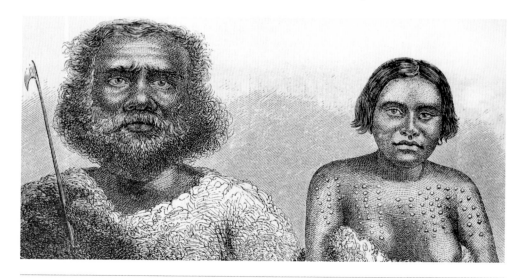

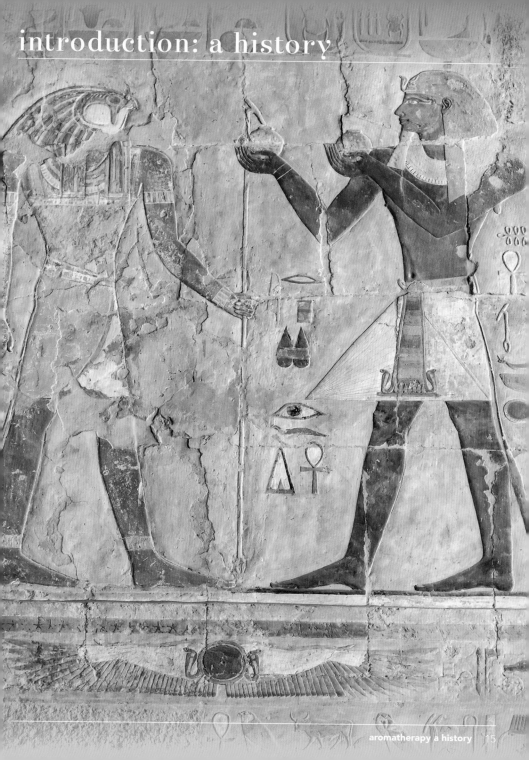

The Aborigines of Australia crushed leaves of the Tea Tree plant and used the paste as a natural antiseptic and disinfectant for thousands of years – a practice which continues to this very day. In the 1920s it was proved that Tea Tree was a much more powerful antiseptic than the most commonly used alternative of the time.

Ancient Egyptians used Cedar and Myrrh for embalming purposes helping to preserve bodies until their discovery thousands of years later.

Jars of Frankincense were found in tombs dating from 3000BC. Formulae were inscribed onto stone tablets, which is how we know so much about what the Egyptians of that time were doing with natural ingredients.

The Nile Valley in Egypt (also known as the 'Cradle of Medicine') was a popular destination for people from other cultures. Many visited this area to gain knowledge and discover more about the use of plants.

The Greeks in particular benefitted from this sharing of knowledge, particularly Hippocrates (from whose name we get the term "Hippocratic Oath").

Hippocrates was a visionary and his work became highly important in the early development of the usage of plants in medicinal treatments. He was a prolific writer on the subject and so helped many others to understand the best ways to use the natural properties of plants and herbs – both at the time and ever since.

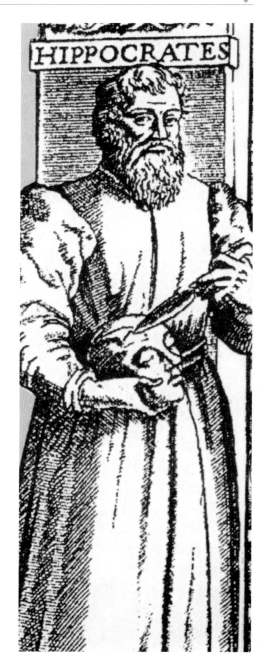

HIPPOCRATES

introduction: a history

Another important name in the fascinating history of Aromatherapy is that of Abd Allah ibn Sina, more commonly known as Avicenna. He spent a lifetime accurately describing 800 plants and their potential uses having been a child prodigy and qualifying as a doctor by the time he was 18.

He also presented exact instructions for massage and he is believed to have discovered (or at least perfected) the process of distillation for producing essential oils – his methods still resonate even today.

There is a deep and varied history of the use of plants and herbs for medical purposes in India and China. Traditional Indian Ayurvedic treatments date back thousands of years, while many of the traditional techniques used for millennia in Chinese medicine are now commonplace around the world – think acupuncture, shiatsu or the use of herbal medicines.

We're all familiar with the concept of a delicious scented bath nowadays. It was the Romans who developed this idea in their public baths. Essential oils were used both in the water and in massage.

Journeys of Knowledge: Europe was comparatively late to embrace the benefits of Aromatherapy. There is little evidence of even basic knowledge or indeed the use of herbal medicine in Western Europe until around the time of the Crusades between the 11th and 13th century.

Knights and soldiers returned from their voyages bringing perfumes, stories and knowledge of new discoveries in the world of natural medicine. Europeans started to experiment with the plants growing in their own countries – Lavender and Rosemary among them.

References to Lavender water and methods of making infused oils can be found in medieval manuscripts.

During the Middle Ages people wore herbal bouquets (known as trussy-mussies) and carried plants to protect themselves against infection. Henry VIII established a charter in 1543 proclaiming the right of herbalists to practise.

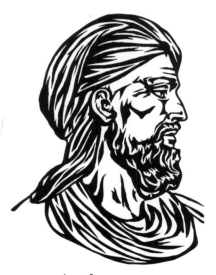

Avicenna

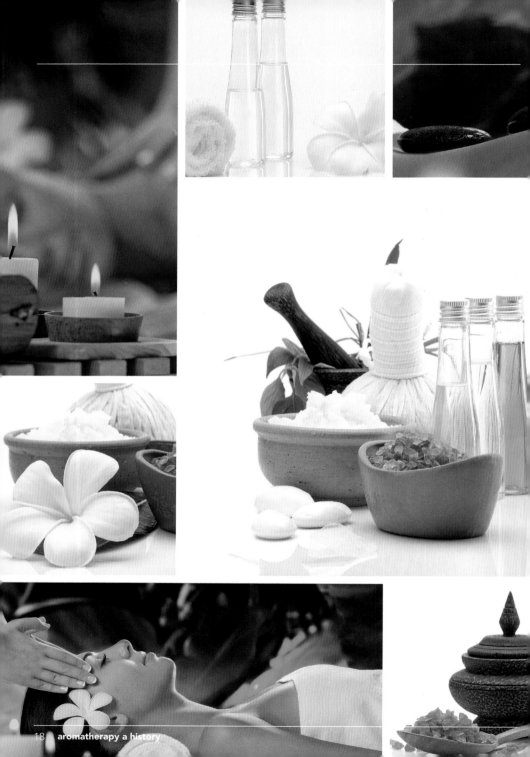

introduction: a history

Developments in theories and practice: Nicholas Culpeper and John Gerard both published books ('The English Physician' & 'The Great Herbal' respectively) on the subject in the 17th century as the knowledge and use of herbal medicine became ever more widespread.

During the 19th century developments in chemistry made it easier to extract oils. Advancements in printing techniques enabled many more books and texts on the subject to be printed. This had an effect in two ways.

The positive effect was that Aromatherapy practices became even more popular. However, it also had what was to become a negative effect in that it became much easier to focus on the individual elements of essential oils.

This ultimately led to the creation of artificial synthetic versions of these elements. These were much cheaper and became more readily available as they were produced on a much larger scale than the natural originals.

Due to the amount of money the companies producing these new synthetic products made, they were able to discredit the very thing that had prompted their success. So, despite thousands of years of tradition and success, herbal medicine was taken less seriously and derided by scientists and the media.

Aromathérapie: In the 1900s a French chemist called René Maurice Gattefossé discovered that Lavender Oil helped burns to heal and also prevented scarring. This happened after he burned his hand while working in the family perfumery business. He sank his hand in to a vat of Lavender and noted the extraordinary results. The Lavender Oil helped his burns to heal and prevented scarring.

As a result, Gattefossé used various oils on the wounds suffered by soldiers in the First World War and saw that the soldiers recovered much quicker than by using conventional means alone.

Gattefossé coined the term "Aromathérapie" and first used the term in a research paper published in 1928. This prompted several other French scientists to continue Gattefossé's research.

Perhaps the most prominent of these was Dr Jean Valnet who broadened research into the effect of essential oils on psychological disorders and also used oils to treat soldiers and combat disease during the Indo-China war between 1948 and 1959.

One of the followers of Valnet's work was Marguerite Maury. An Austrian biochemist, she was responsible for bringing Aromatherapy to the UK. She discovered that essential oils used during massage were easily absorbed into the skin and in the 1940s she set up several Aromatherapy practices.

Her students then set up their own practices and the tradition of Aromatherapy in beauty and massage treatments became firmly established in Britain as a consequence.

Modern Day Aromatherapy:
In 1977 Robert Tisserand published "The Art of Aromatherapy" which concentrated more on the health and clinical therapy benefits of essential oils and plant extracts.

In modern times Aromatherapy has become recognised as a genuinely useful and effective addition or alternative to modern medicine as well as becoming an increasingly vital ingredient in many big name cosmetic and skincare preparations.

People have become more aware of the sometimes dangerous synthetic chemicals used in almost every area of modern medicine and a desire and need for more natural therapies has seen Aromatherapy grow in popularity once again.

Ongoing research has often proved what many millions of people already knew about some essential oils and has shown many of them to be effective natural alternatives. For example, Nottingham Hospital in the UK offers an Aromatherapy service

for women in labour. There are many published articles on the benefits of Aromatherapy in the treatment of cancer.

As with any medical treatment, Aromatherapy does not claim to be some sort of magical cure-all. It is incumbent on us all to look after our own bodies and minds, to take regular exercise to benefit both the physical and mental elements of ourselves and to take responsibility for what we put in to and on to our bodies.

Aromatherapy can be practised at home without expert instruction but care should always be taken when using essential oils. Contraindications should always be carefully checked for each oil before use and if any doubt arises a professional aromatherapist should be consulted.

Medical complaints should normally be treated first and foremost by medical professionals. However, this is a personal choice and if you are interested in a more natural path to health then Aromatherapy can be a fantastic option. Modern Aromatherapy remains an important and, many feel, necessary part of a healthy lifestyle to promote physical and mental well-being.

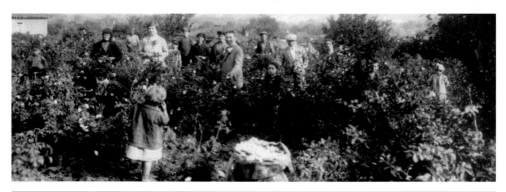

introduction: a history

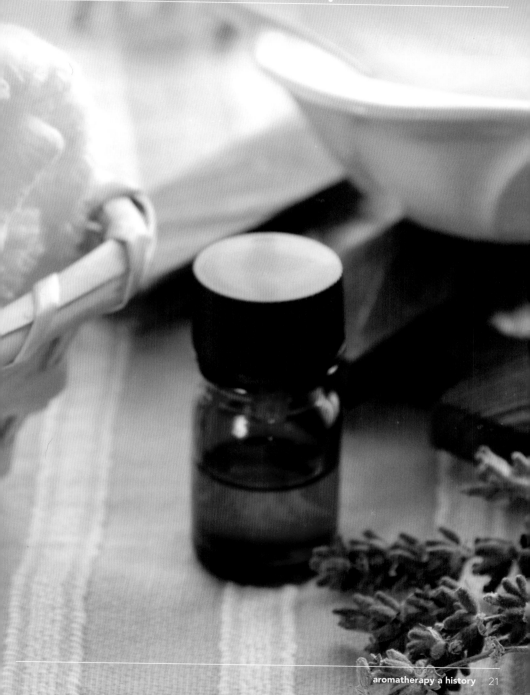

how oils are produced

How to extract essential oils: There are a few different ways to produce essential oils from plants and herbs.

The most common is by steam distillation but this is not suitable for every plant. Citrus oils are normally produced by cold pressing, whilst rare absolutes and concretes are produced via solvent extraction. One of the most commonly asked questions in the world of Aromatherapy is "what is the difference between Absolutes and Essential Oils?".

The basic answer is that Absolutes are normally more potent and stronger than Essential Oils. This is due to the different ways in which the two products are produced. Read on for more detailed information on how different techniques are used to extract the various natural essences.

Steam Distillation: Essential oils have been produced by steam distillation ever since Avicenna perfected the art almost 2000 years ago. A diagram example of steam distillation can be seen opposite. The raw plant material is placed in a chamber before steam is piped in. The steam causes the small sacs containing the essential oil to burst and the oil is then carried out of the chamber in the steam. The steam containing the oils is then cooled in a condensing chamber and returns to a liquid state.

The oil is then separated from the water. The oil is bottled and the water left behind (called a hydrolate) is often sold as flower or floral water. The longer the time allowed to complete this process the better the quality of the oil.

Each oil requires a different temperature of steam to achieve the best results. For example, if the heat is too high then some of the delicate microscopic components of the oil will be damaged or disappear altogether.

Solvent Extraction: Some plants and flowers are too delicate to be steam distilled. In these cases solvent extraction is used to create what is known as an Absolute.

A solvent is added to the plant material. The solvent may be a hydrocarbon or liquefied carbon dioxide. This dissolves the essential oil. The solvent is then evaporated off to leave a combination of plant waxes and essential oils (known as the concrete).

Pure alcohol is then added to the concrete and this extracts the oils from the waxes. The alcohol is then allowed to evaporate leaving behind the Absolute oil.

introduction: production

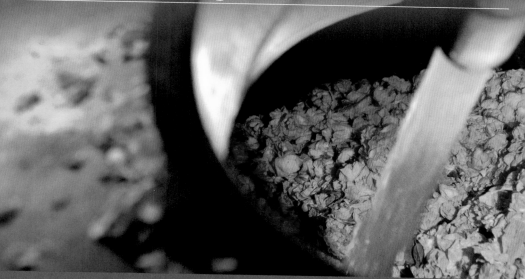

essential oil: steam distillation

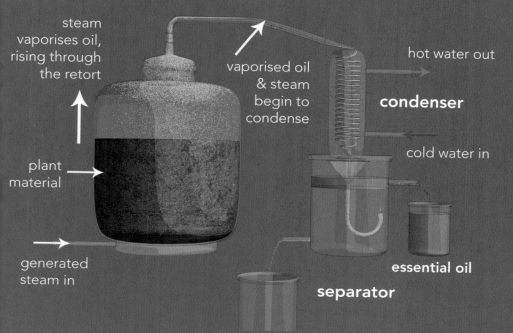

steam vaporises oil, rising through the retort

vaporised oil & steam begin to condense

hot water out

condenser

plant material

cold water in

generated steam in

essential oil

separator

hydrolat/floral water

Cold Pressing (Expression):
Citrus fruits are normally cold pressed to produce the essential oil. If you scratch the rind of an orange, essential oil is the liquid that sprays out. Cold pressing works in a similar way but on a much larger scale. The fruits are passed through machines which score the rind and capture the resulting essential oils.

There are other ways of producing essential oils but the above processes are the 3 most common currently used. Alternative methods include "Folding" (most often used for citrus oils; the plant material is folded 5 or 10 times to squeeze out the essential oil. This produces a highly potent oil which is normally much more expensive than essential oils produced in other ways because of the time and man-hours required).

Another method which is becoming more common is CO_2 extraction. The temperature of the CO_2 is regulated until it reaches 32 degrees Celsius. At this point CO_2 is neither a gas or a liquid but retains the qualities of both. This makes extracting the oil from plants fairly straightforward and because the oil doesn't have to be heated too much the quality of the oil can often be superior.

Again, this is a relatively expensive way of producing essential oils, partly because of the heavy duty equipment required and the fact that a slight error in the temperature or the pressure used to extract the oil can be disastrous. This is why oils produced in this way will also cost more in store.

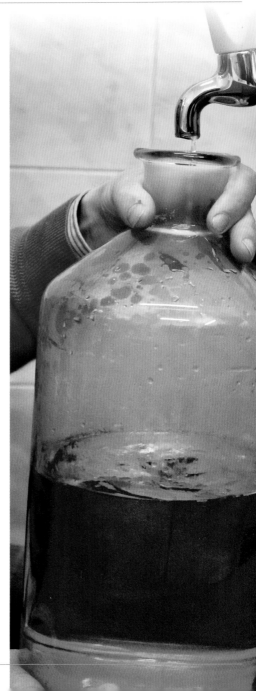

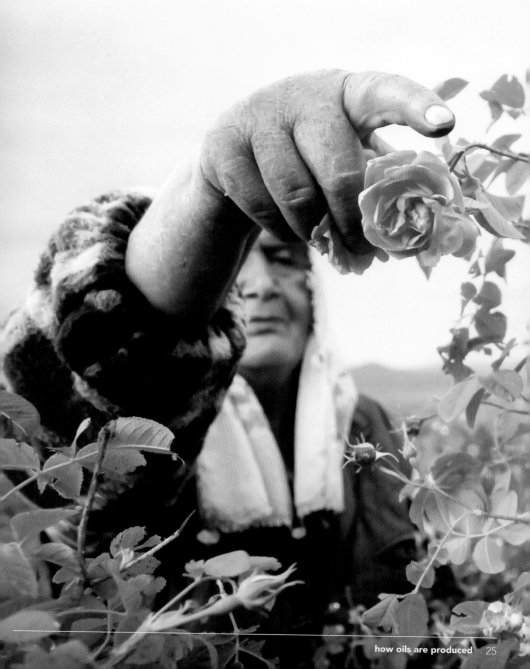

section two

how to use essential oils

how to use essential oils

There are many wonderful ways to use essential oils to benefit health and general well-being. The most popular methods are to burn or vaporise them or add them to a base oil, lotion or cream for massage and skincare treatments.

There's a lot of mystique around essential oils, and whilst care should always be taken, it's actually very simple to use essential oils at home.

In this chapter we will touch on the most commonly employed methods of use and introduce a key system (next to each subtitle) that is used throughout the book. There are general guidelines of how many drops of essential oils to use within each method, however you should refer to the dilution rate chapter for specific cases such as use on children under 12 years old or during pregnancy.

Vaporising (also known as burning) (V):
There are many different types of vaporisers available ranging from simple candle-powered ceramic vaporisers to electric-powered vaporisers and also humidifiers that produce a stream of steam which carries the oil into the air.

When essential oils are vaporised tiny molecules become airborne and enter the body naturally as you breathe. This introduces the essential oils into our bodies via nose and lungs. They are then quickly absorbed into the blood stream allowing the essential oils to start working in the body. They also create a beautiful aroma!

There are hundreds of different candle powered burners available. They are all based around the same basic idea. A bowl is suspended above a candle so the water and the oil(s) are gently warmed. Simply fill the bowl with water and then add up to 8 drops of essential oil.

You'll want to make sure that the device is sturdy and won't wobble or fall over. The bowl shouldn't be too close or too far away from the heat source. Most burners use small nightlight or tea light candles. It's important to ensure that the water doesn't completely evaporate as this can cause the oils to burn which will create an unpleasant acrid smell. Simply top up the water if it looks like it's about to empty.

Electric vaporisers are probably the safest option when children or pets are present or when you want to burn oils late at night or overnight in cases of insomnia. There is no naked flame and they are easy to clean and maintain. They normally consist of a small basin in which the water and oils are placed. This is heated by an element which gently warms the blend. They can normally be left switched on (check the manufacturer's guidelines). Again, 8 drops of oil is a good rule of thumb although more can be added if the vaporiser remains on for a long time.

how to use essential oils

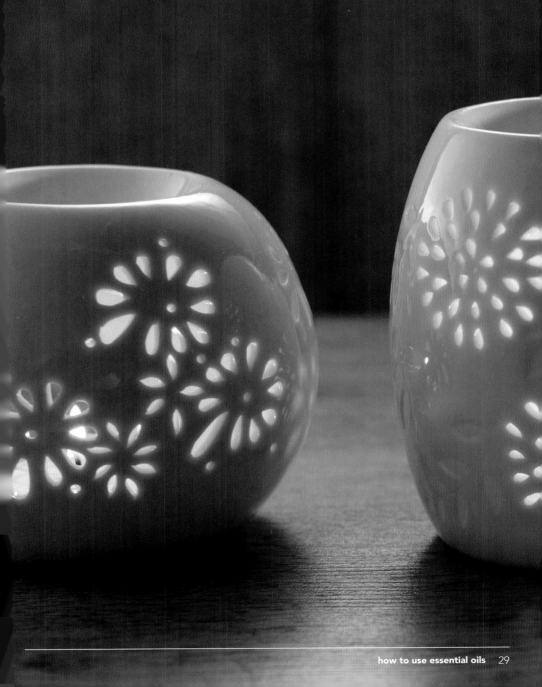

Inhalation (I): Another popular way to benefit from essential oils is via steam inhalation. This is especially effective when dealing with sinus problems or colds etc. and is the best way to alleviate congestion. Simply boil some water, place it in a bowl and then add 2-5 drops of essential oils. Eucalyptus and Tea Tree are most commonly used in this way.

Allow the water to cool for 2-3 minutes or so (freshly boiled water produces steam so hot that it can actually damage the nasal passage), then place a towel over your head so that the steam can travel directly towards your nose. Position your head about 25-30cm above the water. Breathe deeply through your nose for about a minute remembering to keep your eyes shut. If it gets too hot unfurl the towel to cool the face. Avoid scalding the skin with the steam.

Tissues (T): A simple way to benefit from the properties of essential oils is to place a drop or two on a tissue and then inhale regularly. Just add the oils to a tissue, fold in half and then take a deep sniff as often as you feel necessary. The only thing to be aware of is to make sure that the neat essential oils don't come into contact with your skin.

This is perfect for when you wish to feel the benefits of your chosen essential oil quickly and is particularly good if you are on the move. The volatile molecules of the essential oils are absorbed in through the lungs as you deeply sniff the tissue.

Massage treatments (M): Essential oils have been used on the body via application by massage for centuries. An even deeper level of healing can be achieved using this beneficial treatment. Whether working on a localised area or indulging in a full body massage, a bespoke blend can be created for any occasion.

If you create a blend you wish to keep and use another time then make sure to store it in a dark glass bottle – this will help to keep the essential oils vibrant and will ensure that your blend remains useable for a good while.

Creating your own basic massage blends is fairly straightforward. First of all you should check that the essential oil(s) you want to use are safe for application to the skin. You'll need to ensure that the ratio of essential oils to base oil is correct. You can find suggested ratios in the Carrier Oils and Dilution Rates chapters.

The vast majority of essential oils are safe for this purpose. The maximum recommended ratio for most oils is 5% (some are much less – 1-2%. Always check the recommended ratios for each oil before you use them for the first time). For example, for a 5% blend then you'll need 100mls of base oil to which you would add a total maximum of 5mls of essential oils.

So, if you were planning a blend of Chamomile and Lavender for a nice, relaxing massage you would add 2.5mls of each oil to 100mls of base oil.

The most commonly used base oil is Sweet Almond followed by Grapeseed. Add the essential oils to your base oil (preferably in a dark glass bottle as this will help the blend to keep longer)

how to use essential oils

and give it a good shake to ensure it is thoroughly blended.

There are different methods of massage depending on the ailment you are trying to remedy.

Most home massages will be aimed at relaxing the person being massaged. Simply add a few drops of your massage blend to the area of the body you are massaging. Then place a few drops on your hands, rub them together and then start to massage.

You will need to communicate with the person you are massaging to establish how hard or soft they like to be massaged. We'll take a back massage as an example: start at the bottom of the area you are massaging and work upwards. Use both hands and continue to massage until you feel the blend has been sufficiently absorbed by the body. Repeat until your "patient" feels that they've had enough.

If you are massaging the arms or legs then it's generally best to work towards the heart. This encourages the blood flow to circulate much more efficiently and means that you are working with the natural path of the flow of blood rather than against it.

Those mentioned above are very basic massage techniques that are suitable for carrying out a treatment at home. There are many and varied ways that a professional masseuse will be able to offer treatment and plenty of sources in print and on the internet to help you discover new ways to apply essential oils via massage.

Aromatherapy skincare (S): There is an essential oil for pretty much every skin complaint or problem. Whether used for general or therapeutic purposes essential oils are highly beneficial for skincare. They are easily absorbed by the skin to improve the localised area and then deeper into the capillaries within the dermis, into the blood stream.

It's simple to create a blend. Just measure the amount of base ingredient you want to use (cream or lotion for example) and then add the appropriate number of drops of essential oils. Mix thoroughly before each application.

You'll find different recommended dilution rates for the face and body along with guidelines for different age groups in the Dilution Rate chapter. Essential oils are strong and so you should avoid using them on the delicate skin around the eyes.

Generally speaking it's good to use a low dilution rate of around 2-3% for general purpose treatments. Therapeutic treatments may go up to 5%. All the spice oils, Sage and all the citrus oils should be used with great care if being applied to the skin. They should be diluted to a maximum of 1% to 2%.

In both skincare and massage treatments it's advisable to perform a skin patch test before applying the oils to the area to be treated. Simply make up a small amount of the blend at a maximum dilution rate of 2-3% (for example 2-3 drops of essential oil in 5ml of base cream, lotion or carrier oil), apply a few drops to an unobtrusive patch of skin and ideally cover with a plaster. Wait 24 hours to see if any sensitisation occurs. If any adverse reaction is experienced then the oil should not be used.

Occasionally, repeated or overuse of any oil can also lead to sensitisation. If this happens stop using the oil straight away. You may find that you will be able to use the oil again after a while once the body has readjusted.

Hair and scalp treatments (H):
The way to beautiful hair is through a well-nourished and balanced scalp. By using a combination of carrier oils and essential oils it is easy to prepare hair and scalp treatments that can be used once a week for general maintenance or more frequently if treating conditions such as dandruff.

Pick an appropriate base oil for your needs and add your chosen essential oil(s), using a dilution rate of 3% for general use, up to 5% for therapeutic purposes. Mix the blend well and work into the scalp using fingertips in small circular motions. This will encourage circulation within the scalp as well as promoting a feeling of relaxation.

It's good to drape a towel over your shoulders to prevent spillage onto clothes as you smooth the blend along the hair to the tips. To open the cuticle further, it is possible to wrap the hair in a shower cap and/or towel. Leave the treatment on for a minimum of 30 minutes though a longer time span (even overnight) achieves a deeper treatment.

Bathing (B): The time-honoured ritual of bathing for health, cleanliness and relaxation can be enhanced by adding essential oils. If you are experiencing aching muscles and joints after exercise, chills and stuffiness from illness, skin irritations or just wish to unwind, an aromatic bath can make a real difference.

Simply fill the bath to the desired depth and temperature and add up to 8 drops. As the essential oils can 'sit' on the water surface it is best to swish the water to disperse. It is also possible to use milk as a dispersing ingredient, just add your 8 drops to a little milk and add to the bath water.

During bathing the essential oils absorb through the skin, into the system and imbue their therapeutic properties. Other popular additions to baths include Dead Sea salt, Epsom salts, flower petals or herbs.

Essential oils can also be used to great effect in the shower by dripping the oils onto a flannel or sponge and rubbing over the body. The stream of water instantly dilutes the oils whilst the warmth of the water creates a beautifully enveloping steam treatment.

Alternatively a blend can be added to a carrier oil and applied over the body before stepping into the shower (this technique can be used before bathing also). The skin is left richly moisturised. Be careful though – the oils will create a very slippery floor as they run off your body!

Another lovely way to introduce essential oils into your system is to submerge your feet into a bowl of warm water. The soles of the feet contain thousands of nerve endings which relate to different parts of the body and are one of the most readily 'absorbent' areas of your whole body.

Just fill a stable-bottomed bowl (big enough to put both your feet in) with warm water and add up to 5 drops of essential oils dispersing in the same manner as bathing. Remember to have a towel to dry your feet close by. You might also like to create a matching foot lotion for use after the soak.

Compresses (C): Compresses are most commonly used in cases of aches and sprains and are easy to create by swishing 5-6 drops of essential oil into hot or cold water.

Choose the temperature which will be most beneficial to the ailment. Cold compresses are best for headaches and also when treating twists or sprains as this will help to restrict any swelling or inflammation. Hot compresses are good for stiff and achy muscles.

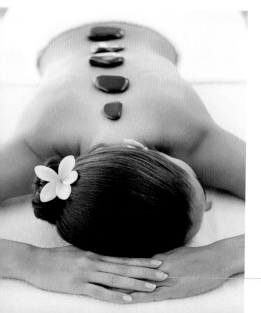

Submerge a flannel, wring out and apply to the troubled location. This process can be repeated several times.

Around the house and office:
Essential oils are incredibly useful through the home and even workspaces. Many have antibacterial and anti-fungal properties which can be used in kitchens and bathrooms. Just add a few drops to hot water along with a little soap to disinfect work surfaces, sinks, tiles and baths.

Most of the citrus oils – particularly Lime and Lemon – make a great alternative to chemical-packed cleaning products. Simply dilute 5-10 drops of each in boiled water that has been allowed to cool and use to clean tops and work surfaces in the same way you would your normal cleaner.

Lemon is also great for cleaning windows and mirrors.

Diluted Tea Tree is a great way to clean away patches of mould or mildew and will also help to prevent it recurring as quickly as it might otherwise.

Lavender is another great oil to use for cleaning. You can either make up your own blend or simply add it to your existing washing liquid to enhance the antiseptic and antibacterial action.

There are many other ways in which essential oils can be used. A quick search on the internet will produce hundreds of recipes using dozens of different techniques so you will be able to quickly find a solution to most problems.

dilution rates

dilution rates

Essential oils are incredibly potent and should always be diluted before applying to the skin. The maximum dilution rate is 5% essential oil in a carrier oil or base product (such as a cream or shampoo). However it is advisable to use a dilution rate of 3% on most occasions as a stronger treatment does not equate to a better or more effective treatment. You may find that chronic cases require the maximum dilution of 5% though careful observation of results should be noted.

For massage: 3% – 3 drops to each 5ml of carrier oils.

Facial Application: 1% maximum – 1 drop to each 5ml of carrier oil or cream.

Children: Not for use under 3 years old unless under the guidance of a qualified aromatherapist.

Over 3 to 7 years old – 0.5%, 1 drop to 10mls of base product.

Over 7 to 12 years old – 1% to 1.5%, as indicated for facial applications 12 years old and above – as directed for adult use.

Pregnancy:

First trimester:	Inadvisable to use any essential oils
Second trimester:	1%
Third trimester:	2%

Please take note of cautions at the bottom of each essential oil page. Some oils can encourage menstrual bleeding and so should be avoided completely during the entire pregnancy.

Essential Oil minimum to maximum drops	ml of base preparation	
0 to 1	1	20 drops = 1ml
2 to 5	5	40 drops = 2ml
4 to 10	10	60 drops = 3ml
6 to 15	15	
8 to 20	20	5ml = 1tsp
10 to 25	25	10ml = 1dsp
12 to 30	30	15ml = 1tbsp

dilution rates

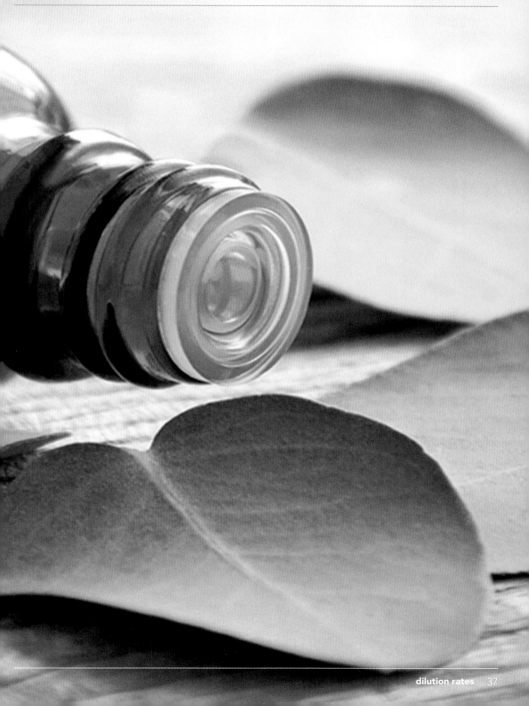

section four

essential oils

bergamot

Citrus bergamia: *From the plant family Rutaceae.*

Originates from tropical Asia but is historically most popular in Italy where the oil is almost exclusively produced nowadays.

The oil is produced by expression of the peel of the fruit. It's often then rectified to remove the furocoumarins (chemicals naturally produced by the plant which can cause phototoxicity).

Properties claimed for Bergamot include: Analgesic, antiseptic, antiviral, cooling, relaxing, sedative, laxative, vermifuge and uplifting.

Summary: Bergamot is regarded as an uplifting and cheering oil which is also antiseptic and so used for treating many skin conditions.

History: The tree is named after the small town of Bergamo in Northern Italy where the fruits of the tree were originally cultivated. The fruits have been used for hundreds of years in Italy but were pretty much unknown elsewhere because the fruit was not exported to other countries until relatively recently. The Italians used Bergamot in the treatment of malaria, perhaps because of its antiviral, relaxing and sedative properties.

Bergamot forms the base flavour in Earl Grey and Lady Grey teas and is often used in confectionery and marmalades (especially in Italy). It's used in many perfumes as well as in commercially produced skincare creams.

Usage & Methods of Application: When blended in massage Bergamot is commonly used for various skin conditions including eczema, acne and psoriasis. It can also be used to relieve excessive flatulence, colic and digestive problems and may also assist in regulating the appetite. Because of its cooling action Bergamot can also be useful in lessening the effect of feverish conditions.

Aromatherapists use Bergamot to help to relieve the symptoms of colds and flu, to treat inflammatory problems such as tonsillitis or sore throats and it has also been used successfully to treat cystitis or urethritis as it is thought to have a powerful effect on problems in the urinary tract.

Bergamot is one of the most commonly used oils to treat psychological issues as it's regarded as a very good uplifting oil and relaxing oil. People suffering from depression brought on by stress are often advised to burn or vaporise Bergamot because of these properties.

It's also used as an antiviral oil with particular potency against the herpes simplex virus which causes cold sores. It's used alone or blended with Geranium

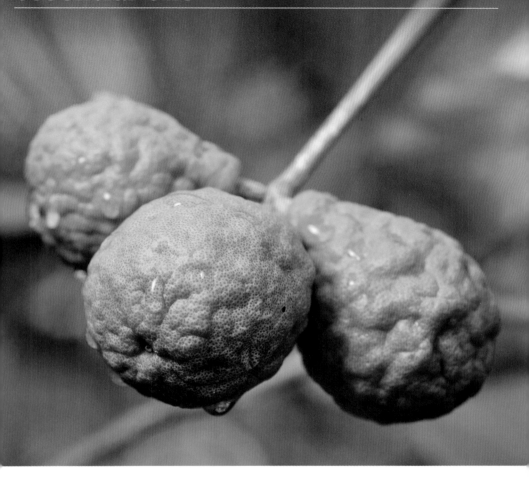

as it can stop cold sores developing if used when the first ominous tingle is felt.

Blends well with: Most essential oils blend well with one another. You may find that Bergamot blends especially well with Black Pepper, Clary Sage, Cypress, Frankincense, Geranium, Jasmine, Mandarin, Nutmeg, Orange, Rosemary, Sandalwood, Vetiver and Ylang Ylang.

Toxicity & safety: Unadulterated Bergamot oil contains Bergaptene and so should not be used before or during a spell in the sun as it will dramatically increase the likelihood of sunburn.

Most commercially available Bergamot oils have been rectified to remove this, however care should still be taken in these circumstances. Always check with your supplier as to whether the oil has been rectified.

cedarwood atlas

Cedrus atlantica: *From the plant family Pinaceae.*
Native to the Atlas Mountains of Algeria and Morocco.
The oil is obtained by steam distillation of the bark of the tree.
Properties claimed for Cedarwood Atlas include: Antiseptic, antifungal, astringent, diuretic, expectorant, nervine, sedative and tonic.

Summary: One of the more popular essential oils for men thanks to its sweet and woody aroma, Cedarwood Atlas is also used to treat acne and other skin complaints.

History: Believed to be one of the first essential oils ever to be produced, records from ancient times suggest that the oil and the wood were used for incense as well as in medicine and cosmetics.

The wood was used as a material for buildings and also for furniture. The natural odour of the wood was considered to repel moths and other insects. It's still used in some parts of the world today to make clothes hangers for the same reason.

Cedarwood Atlas oil was hugely popular with the Ancient Egyptians. It was one of the oils used for embalming purposes as well as for fumigation. Other historical uses include as a cure for baldness, to treat bronchial and urinary tract infections and in treatments for the skin.

Tibetans still use the oil as a temple incense and it's commonly found in their traditional medicines. Today it's found as a fragrance (often as a fixative) in cosmetics and perfumes as well as in soaps and detergents.

Usage & methods of application: When blended in a base oil or lotion Cedarwood Atlas is often used in the treatment of acne, dermatitis, eczema, fungal infections and other skin complaints. It may also be used to soothe the symptoms of arthritis and rheumatism and to ease problems associated with bronchitis, excessive catarrh and coughs. It's sometimes included in relaxing massage blends to help with nervous tension and other stress-related symptoms.

It can be added to a base shampoo or conditioner to help with greasy hair, dandruff and there are even those who believe it can help to reduce baldness.

When burned or vaporised it's often added to blends for its sweet and woody aroma as well as its calming and stress-releasing properties.

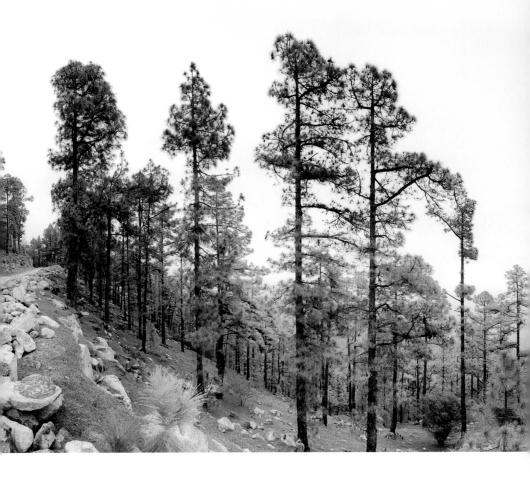

This same aroma makes it very popular in blends to be used by men.

Blends well with: Most essential oils blend well with one another. You may find that Cedarwood Atlas blends especially well with Rosewood, Bergamot, Cypress, Cassia, Jasmin, Juniper, Neroli, Clary Sage, Vetivert, Rosemary and Ylang Ylang.

Toxicity & safety: Non-toxic, non-sensitising and non-irritant. However, Cedarwood Atlas should be avoided by pregnant and nursing mothers.

chamomile roman

Anthemis nobilis: From the plant family Asteraceae.

Originally from southern and western Europe and now naturalised to North America. Cultivated in the UK, Belgium, the USA, France and Italy.

Obtained by steam distillation of the dried flowering heads of the plant.

Properties claimed for Chamomile Roman include: Analgesic, antispasmodic, anti-inflammatory, bactericidal, carminative, digestive, emmenagogue, hypnotic, sedative and tonic.

Summary: Perhaps one of the most well-known of all the essential oils, Chamomile comes in several different varieties although the most commonly used are Roman and Matricaria (German). It has a plethora of potential uses but is probably most used for its ability to calm and soothe.

History: Chamomile has a long and rich medicinal history. It's been known in Europe and the Mediterranean for over 2000 years and was used by the ancient Egyptians. It was also one of the nine sacred herbs of the Saxons and is well regarded by gardeners as it promotes the health of nearby plants.

The Egyptians used it to treat acute fever while the Romans burned it as incense and used it to flavour drinks. The name "Roman" came about in the 19th century when a plant collector discovered it growing in the Coliseum in Rome.

In modern times it can be found in many pharmaceutical ointments, both for its antiseptic and its calming qualities. It's used extensively in cosmetics, soaps, detergents, perfumes and hair and bath products.

Usage & methods of application: Chamomile Roman is often found in Aromatherapy massage blends aimed at treating acne, allergy rashes, boils, burns, cuts and abrasions, chilblains, dermatitis, eczema, inflammations, insect bites and stings and sensitive skin. It's also used to alleviate the symptoms of arthritis, swollen joints, rheumatism and muscular pain.

When burned or vaporised it may help to relieve headaches, insomnia, nervous tension and stress-related issues.

Blends well with: Essential oils generally blend well with one another. You may find that Chamomile Roman blends especially well with Bergamot, Clary Sage, Lavender, Geranium, Jasmine, Tea Tree, Grapefruit, Rose, Lemon and Ylang Ylang.

Toxicity & safety: Chamomile Roman is non-toxic and non-irritant although it may cause dermatitis in some people if used incorrectly or if they are allergic to Ragwort. Always dilute to 5% or less before application to the skin.

essential oils

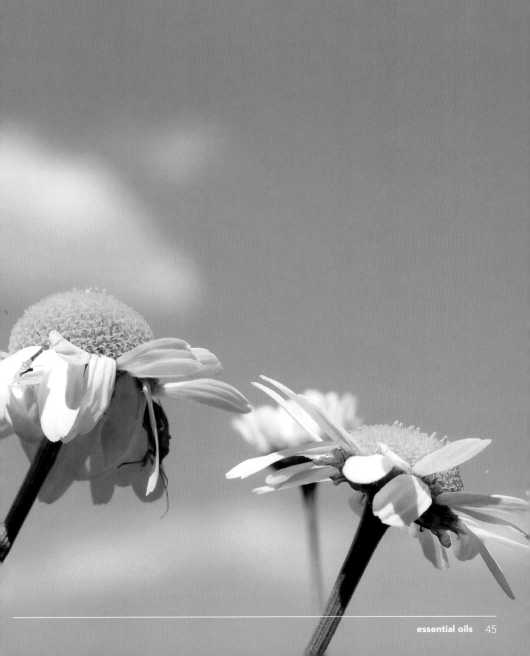

cinnamon

Cinnamomum zeylanicum: From the plant family Lauraceae. Originally from Madagascar and south east Asia. Obtained by steam distillation of the leaves of the plant. Properties claimed for Cinnamon essential oil include: Analgesic, antiseptic, antispasmodic, aphrodisiac, astringent, insecticide, stimulant and tonic.

Summary: Cinnamon leaf oil is a strong oil which should always be used with caution and in a very low dilution if being applied to the skin. It has many potential uses such as soothing cramps, adding a warming effect to massage blends and is also considered to be an aphrodisiac.

History: Cinnamon has long been one of the most traded spices with a traceable history stretching back over hundreds of years. The Ancient Egyptians used it for embalming potions, perfumes, oils and incense. It is recorded that 350g of Cinnamon traded for more than 1000 Denares at the time of the 1st Century – that's about the equivalent of 5KG of silver at the time. It even gets a mention in the Old Testament.

The Arabs controlled the supply of many spices including Cinnamon until around 1500AD before the Portuguese, the Dutch, the French and even the British had a go at grabbing their share of the market over the next few hundred years.

Nowadays all commercially available Cinnamon is grown on plantations meaning that it's still allowed to grow wild in many countries. The advantage of plantation growing is that the trees are regularly coppiced leading to a higher yield from each tree year after year.

The oil is used for its therapeutic and fragrant properties in many toothpastes, mouthwashes, nasal sprays, cough syrups and dental preparations as well as in soaps, cosmetics, toiletries and perfumes. It's also commonly found in food flavourings, especially soft and alcoholic drinks.

Usage & methods of application: Cinnamon can be used on the skin but must always be very well diluted (1-2% max) as it can be an irritant to the skin as well as the mucous membrane. It's used in massage to improve circulation and to help with the symptoms of rheumatism. It may also be used as a rub for the stomach to help with digestive problems or stomach cramps.

It's often burned or vaporised (again in small amounts) to protect against airborne viruses and germs and also to alleviate the symptoms of colds and flu as well as helping with nervous exhaustion and stress-related symptoms.

essential oils

Blends well with: Most essential oils blend well with one another. You may find that Cinnamon blends especially well with Benzoin, Clove, Coriander, Cardamom, Frankincense, Ginger, Grapefruit, Lavender, Rosemary and Thyme.

Toxicity & safety: Cinnamon should never be used by pregnant or nursing mothers due to its emmenagogue properties. It should always be very well diluted before use on the skin as it can be an irritant and should be used in low doses in burners or vaporisers because of the high eugenol content of the oil.

citronella

Cymbopogon Winterianus: From the plant family Poaceae.

The plant is native to Sri Lanka but grows well in any warm and temperate climate. China has become a major grower and distiller of Citronella.

The essential oil is obtained by steam distillation of the grass leaves.

Properties claimed for Citronella oil include: Antiseptic, bactericidal, deodorant, diaphoretic, insecticide, parasitic, tonic and stimulant.

Summary: Citronella is well known for its ability to repel insects but it also has plenty of other uses as well. It's not particularly well known for use in Aromatherapy but can be used for a variety of ailments.

History: Citronella has been used for centuries as a natural insect repellent. It's also been used as a medicinal oil for hundreds of years, particularly in China where it's used to treat rheumatism and arthritis.

Research has also shown that Citronella contains strong antifungal properties.

Usage & methods of application: Citronella is mainly found as an ingredient in candles, perfumery, detergents and soaps. It is little used in Aromatherapy but is useful for adulterating other oils. There are some claims that it's a good oil to use in massage blends for rheumatism.

Its antiseptic and bactericidal properties mean it's occasionally used (on its own or blended with others) to fight cold and flu symptoms.

Citronella may be added to a burner or vaporiser to ward off airborne viruses and germs. You may also find that it assists in lifting the spirits and any feeling of weakness. According to EU legislation we are not allowed to say that it's good for repelling insects but if you are one of the thousands of people who use it for this purpose then there is no reason to stop doing so.

When added to massage blends Citronella is thought to assist in relieving muscular aches and pains. It may also be useful in combating smelly and excessively sweaty feet. It's also sometimes used in skin care preparations for oily skin.

Citronella has been shown as a very useful oil to use in conjunction with pets. Research has shown that the oil is effective in stopping dogs from persistent barking when used in a Citronella collar. The collar contains a microphone and when the dog barks a spray of Citronella is released. The dog finds this so repellent that it quickly learns to stop barking. This is a natural and less unpleasant treatment than the electric shock collars often used in this scenario.

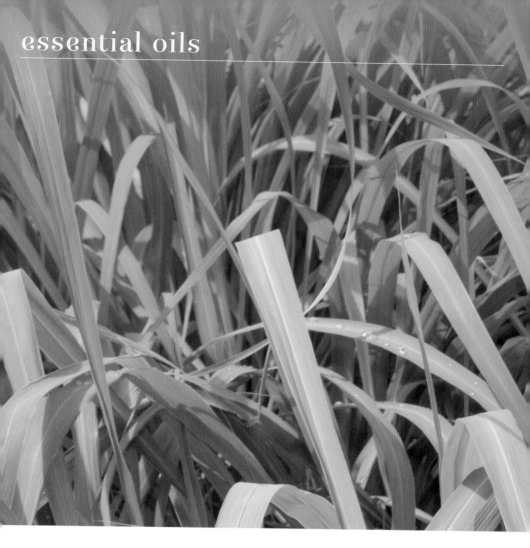

There is also evidence that a spray of Citronella can stop pets from destroying household items such as furniture.

Blends well with: Essential oils generally blend well with one another. You may find that Citronella blends particularly well with Benzoin, Clove, Coriander, Cardamom, Frankincense, Ginger, Grapefruit, Lavender, Rosemary and Thyme.

Toxicity and safety: Citronella should not be used by anyone with sensitive skin and as with any natural product, a skin patch test before full usage is always advised. It's phototoxic so shouldn't be used immediately before, after or during time spent in the sun.

clary sage

Salvia sclarea: *From the plant family Lamiaceae (Labiatae).*
Native to Italy, Syria and southern France but grows well wherever the soil is dry enough.
Obtained by steam distillation of the flowering tops and foliage of the plant.
Properties claimed for Clary Sage Oil include: Anti-inflammatory, antispasmodic, relaxing, sedative, tonic, uplifting and hypotensive.

Summary: Clary Sage is a soothing, calming and relaxing oil with good uplifting properties too.

History: Clary Sage has a long history stretching back to medieval times. Authors of the time named it "Clear Eye" and claimed that it would heal all eye disorders. Nicholas Culpeper was more specific, explaining that the sticky mucilage obtained from the seeds would clear any small detritus from the eye lids. This usage continued in to the Middle Ages when the herb became known as "Oculus Christi" (Eyes of Christ).

In the sixteenth century brewers in Britain used Clary Sage instead of Hops to produce an ale with an heightened intoxicating effect. This soon fell out of favour due to the terrible hangovers suffered by those who drank it!

Usage & methods of application: In massage Clary Sage is used to alleviate oily skin, relax muscles (including cramps and spasms) and to relieve muscle fatigue. It's regarded as an especially good oil for female maladies and is often found in blends aimed at alleviating the symptoms of PMT and the menopause.

In skincare it's often blended with a cream or lotion to offer a general boost to the complexion – especially for those with wrinkled, inflamed skin or acne.

When burned or vaporised it's used to lift the spirits and promote a feeling of well-being, soothe nervous tension or panic and is generally regarded as a calming oil. Additionally it is thought to calm headaches or migraines and may have a positive effect on asthma and other respiratory disorders. Furthermore it's used as a general tonic to strengthen the immune system which makes it a popular oil to use with those who are weak or recovering from illness or surgery etc.

Toxicity & safety: Clary Sage is a non-toxic, non-sensitising and non-irritant but should be avoided by pregnant women and those suffering from estrogen related disorders. It should be avoided after drinking alcohol as it can exacerbate the effects of drinking. Overuse can cause headaches and giddiness and may even raise blood pressure.

essential oils

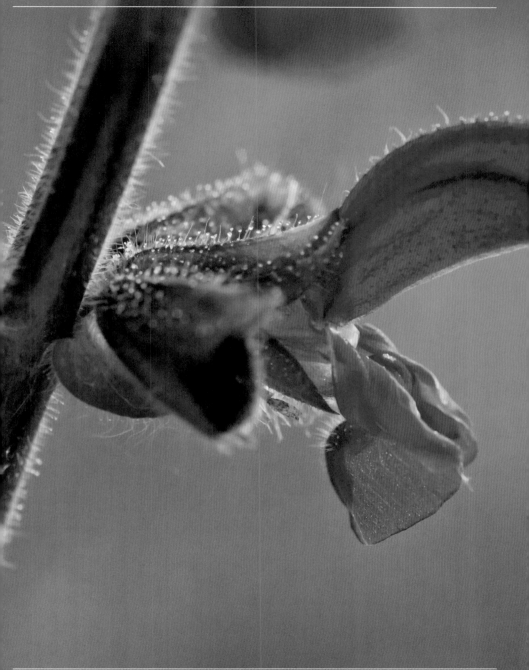

clove

Eugenia caryophyllus: From the plant family Myrtaceae.

Thought to be native to Indonesia but now found worldwide, especially in the Philippines and Madagascar.

The oil is obtained by steam distillation of the dried buds of the plant.

Properties claimed for Clove essential oil include: Antibiotic, antihistaminic, antineuralgic, anti-oxidant, antiseptic, antiviral, aphrodisiac, carminative, counter-irritant, expectorant, and stimulant.

Summary: It's important to ensure that you are using Clove Bud oil rather than the leaf or stem oil which are powerful skin irritants due to the high levels of eugenol found within. Perhaps best known for reducing the pain of toothache, Clove is however a versatile oil with varied potential applications.

History: It's thought that Cloves have been used in Chinese medicine since as far back as 600AD and were prevalent in Ayurvedic medicine too. It's long been a popular spice in the West after being introduced via the Spice Routes. In Asia garlands of Clove flowers are placed around the necks of children to ward off evil spirits (this may be connected with the ability of the oil to repel insects).

In Indonesia Clove is used to flavour cigarettes and it has been used by various cultures around the world to calm upset stomachs and to clear intestinal worms.

Nowadays Clove can be found in dental preparations (many dentists now use diluted Clove in the spray they use to clear the mouth of any detritus and reduce the risk of infections during tooth extractions and other dental procedures).

It's used in toothpastes, soaps, toiletries, cosmetics and perfumes (mainly as a fragrance compound). It's used in the production of many foods and drinks both soft and alcoholic. Furthermore it can be found in inks, glue and varnish.

Usage & methods of application: Used in massage Clove should be very well diluted (to 1% maximum) before application to the skin. It's used in cases of acne, athlete's foot, bruises, burns, cuts and wounds. It can also be found in massage blends aimed at alleviating the symptoms of arthritis, rheumatism and sprains.

When burned or vaporised it is used to relieve the symptoms of asthma and bronchitis.

It's never advisable to use any essential oil neat but hundreds of thousands of people use Clove oil to alleviate the pain

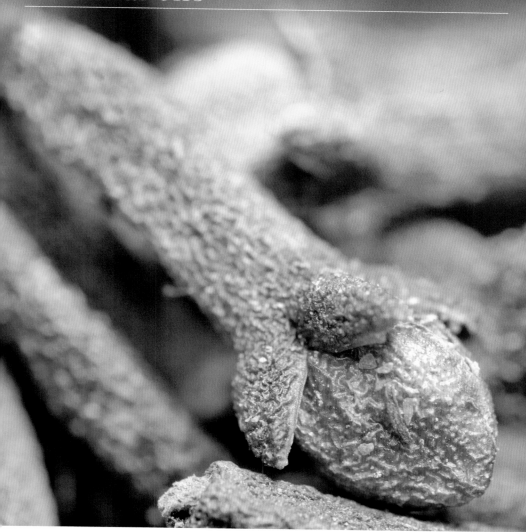

of toothache so that is a decision for the individual.

Blends well with: Essential oils generally blend well with one another. You may find that Clove oil blends particularly well with Benzoin, Cinnamon, Ginger, Sandalwood, Clary Sage, Lavender and Basil.

Toxicity & safety: Clove bud may cause skin and mucous membrane irritation and may lead to dermatitis in some individuals if used incorrectly. Clove oil should be avoided during pregnancy and should not be used on children under 16.

cypress

Cupressus Sempervirens: *From the plant family Cupressaceae.*
The plant is found in Mediterranean countries and parts of North Africa.
The oil is obtained by steam distillation of the leaves of the plant.
Properties claimed for Cypress oil include: Antispasmodic, astringent,
haemostatic, diuretic, tonic and uplifting.

Summary: Cypress can help to control the production of liquids in the body so it's often used to help with excess sweat or body oils, fluid retention and heavy menstrual bleeding. It's commonly found in preparations aimed at sweaty and smelly feet.

History: Another oil with a long history. It's been used in Chinese medicine for thousands of years to control excess sweat amongst other applications. It's been associated with grief and death since the Ancient Egyptians and the Romans dedicated the tree to their gods of death. This is thought to be because the tree is an evergreen and so was linked with eternal life or life after death. It's commonly used to comfort people in times of grief. It's also thought that the cross on which Jesus was crucified was made from Cypress wood.

In modern times Cypress is used in some pharmaceutical products and as a fragrance in colognes, perfumes and after-shaves.

Usage & methods of application:
When applied via massage Cypress is used for a plethora of conditions. These include oily and over hydrated skin, excessive perspiration (particularly the feet), varicose veins, cellulitis, muscular cramp, poor circulation and rheumatism.

It's also thought to act on the bronchial system so can be helpful in cases of asthma, bronchitis and persistent coughs. It can also help to heal broken capillaries – this, combined with the ability to discourage fluid retention makes it a popular oil in blends aimed at relieving the symptoms of the menopause.

When burned or vaporised Cypress is often used during times of grief. It doesn't promise to make grief disappear, rather to help one gain a sense of perspective after the loss of a special one.

The same properties that make it good in massage for the bronchial system also apply when the oil is burned and it's also used in a preventative manner to protect against bugs and viruses.

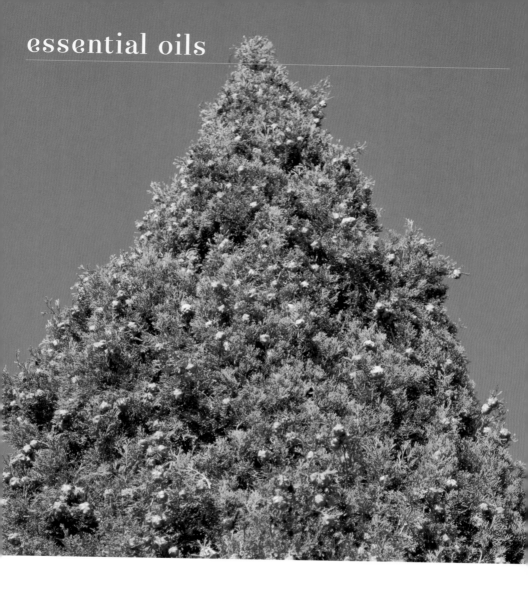

Cypress has good deodorising properties and a masculine, woody aroma so is often found in preparations aimed at men.

Blends well with: You may find that Cypress blends particularly well with Clary Sage, Lavender, Bergamot, Juniperberry, Pine, Rosemary, Frankincense, Sandalwood and the Citrus oils.

Toxicity & safety: Cypress is generally considered to be non-toxic and non-sensitising. However, care should be taken if you are pregnant.

eucalyptus

Eucalyptus globulus: From the plant family Myrtaceae.

Originally found in Tasmania and Australia but nowadays can also be found in countries around the Mediterranean.

The oil is made from the leaves and twigs of the tree.

Extracted by steam distillation.

Properties claimed for Eucalyptus Oil include: Analgesic, antiseptic, antispasmodic, antiviral, depurative, expectorant, prophylactic, stimulant and uplifting.

Summary: Eucalyptus is regarded as a great oil for strengthening the immune system and so is thought to protect the whole body from viruses and disease. It was first discovered by westerners in 1788 but had been used by Australian Aborigines for many centuries before that.

History: Eucalyptus has been used by Australian Aborigines for thousands of years. They used it principally to treat coughs and colds and used a Eucalyptus gum to combat diarrhoea.

Westerners became aware of the oil after the arrival of the First Fleet to Australia in 1788. John White, the Surgeon General for the voyage, noted the olfactory oil in Eucalyptus and a sample was sent over to England for testing. The results of the test showed that the oil was much better at treating coughs and colds than the Peppermint oil that was in favour at the time.

Despite the success of the tests Eucalyptus wasn't exploited to the fullness of its potential until 70 or so years later. Joseph Bosisto was a Victorian pharmacist who qualified in England before moving to Australia. He initially moved to Victoria in 1851 to search for gold but instead set up a pharmacy before commencing production of Eucalyptus oil a year later. He soon set up 4 distilleries to supply local demand for the oil.

In 1865 Bosisto began exporting the oil overseas with the help of Alfred Delton and Frederick Grimwade. Together with some other men they set up a company and over the next 60 years or so they exported hundreds of kilos of the oil all over the world.

Australia was the main producer and exporter of the oil until around 1950 when Mediterranean countries also started producing the oil. These countries were able to supply the oil at cheaper prices due to the lower transport costs etc and the Australian monopoly on the trade was broken. In modern times the oil is

essential oils

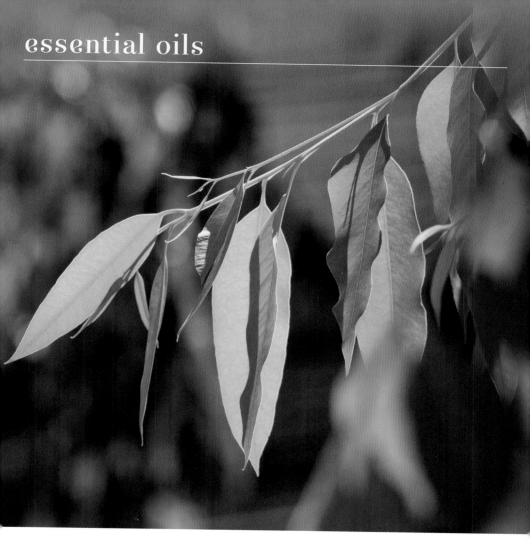

produced by many countries around the world including China. It's thought that around 3000 tonnes of Eucalyptus Oil are consumed in one way or another every year.

Nowadays Eucalyptus is found in a myriad of medicinal products such as cough lozenges, gargles, toothpastes, moistening oils and lotions, inhalation sprays and soaps. You'll also find it in household disinfectants and industrial solvents.

Usage & methods of application:
Eucalyptus has long been recognised for its ability to clear congestion and lessen the symptoms of coughs and colds. When inhaled or burned the antiseptic properties of the oil work to clear infection while the bronchial tubes and nasal passages are also cleared making breathing much easier.

It's also vaporised in saunas and used in massage oils (its anti-inflammatory properties are especially effective for athletes before and after exercise or competition to keep muscles in good working order).

The primary way to use Eucalyptus at home is simply to sniff it straight from the bottle or to place a few drops in your favourite burner or vaporiser. Because it's so good at boosting the immune system it's a great oil to keep handy – you can sniff it once or twice a day to ward off infections and colds etc.

Its clearing properties also make it a good oil for alleviating asthma (although it should not be used during an asthma attack – it's used to improve the overall ability of the body to deal with asthma), sinusitis, bronchitis and other bugs that cause congestion.

It's a natural antiseptic and has germicidal properties which make it good for use on wounds, cuts, ulcers, insect bites and stings and other skin abrasions. We would always recommend that a professional aromatherapist is consulted before using oils on the skin or cuts etc without dilution. A safer way to apply the oil would be to blend it in a carrier oil such as Sweet Almond or Grapeseed before it's put on the skin.

In massage Eucalyptus is used for treating muscular aches and pains and so is often recommended for those suffering from rheumatism, lumbago, sprained ligaments or tendons, stiff muscles and fibrosis. Dilute to 5% or less in a carrier oil and massage the affected area in a circular motion.

When added to a base cream or lotion Eucalyptus is commonly found in blends aimed at easing skin eruptions, oily skin, acne and as a relieving lotion for chicken pox.

It's also a stimulating oil which is often burned or vaporised to help to lift the mood and banish feelings of mental tiredness. It's also often used to treat stress, depression and other mental disorders.

Around the house, Eucalyptus can be added to your laundry in order to provide a lovely fresh feeling to the finished washing. This makes even more sense when you take in to account the deodorising and antiseptic properties of the oil. It makes a great room freshener, especially during times when there are bugs in the house as it not only clears the atmosphere but can also kill airborne germs and viruses.

If you're lucky enough to have a spa or home sauna then you can add Eucalyptus to these too – the rest of us can add a couple of drops to a tablespoon of milk to help it disperse in a lovely warm bath.

Blends well with: All essential oils generally blend well with one another. You may find that Eucalyptus blends particularly well with Benzoin, Thyme, Lavender, Lemongrass, Lemon and Pine.

Toxicity and safety: Eucalyptus oil should never be taken internally unless under the close supervision of a qualified professional aromatherapist. People with high blood pressure and epilepsy should avoid using this oil altogether. Overuse of this oil may cause headaches in rare cases.

essential oils

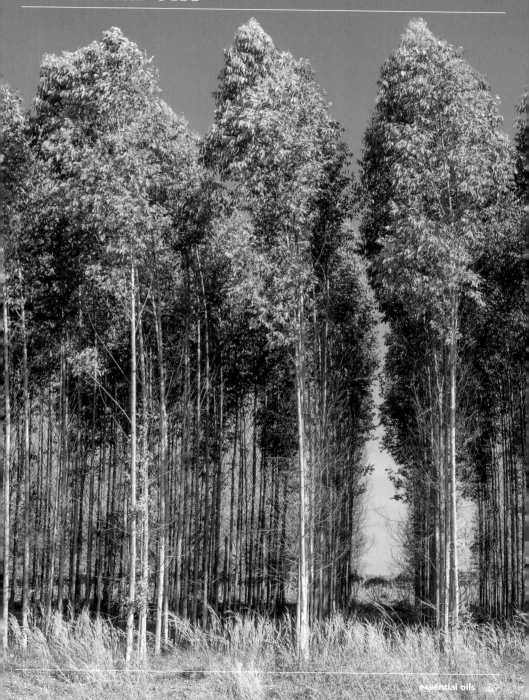

fennel

Foeniculum vulgare: From the plant family Apiaceae (Umbelliferae).
Found the throughout Europe but particularly Mediterranean countries
such as Greece, France and Italy. It seems to prefer growing by the sea.
The essential oil is obtained by steam distillation of the crushed Fennel seeds.
Properties claimed for Fennel essential oil include: Antiseptic,
antispasmodic, carminative, diuretic, galactagogue, emmenagogue,
laxative, antimicrobial and tonic.

Summary: It's important to ascertain that you are buying Sweet Fennel rather than the bitter version. Bitter fennel is considered to be too toxic for use in aromatherapy. Sweet Fennel is a natural diuretic so is often used to purge the body and reduce flatulence, water retention or to ease constipation. It's a powerful oil which should always be used with care.

History: Another plant with a long history. In AD23 it was recorded that serpents rubbed themselves against Fennel. It was thought at the time that this was to improve their eyesight. King Edward I of England mentioned buying Fennel seeds in a journal in 1281 and the Roman army used to eat Fennel seeds to curb hunger pangs and increase courage on their long marches.

In Medieval times it was believed that hanging Fennel seeds on your door would keep evil spirits away and as late as the 17th century William Coles opined that Fennel was a hunger suppressant.

In modern times Fennel can be found in cough drops, lozenges and laxative and carminative preparations. It's commonly found as a flavouring in food, drinks (especially alcoholic drinks such as brandy and liqueurs). You'll also come across it

in soaps, perfumes and toiletries and it's used as a masking agent in room sprays, insecticides and industrial products.

Usage & methods of application: Aromatherapists will often use Fennel in massage blends to be used on bruised, dull, oily and mature skin. It's also used in cases of cellulitis, obesity and rheumatism. It can also be used in a massage around the bowel and intestine area to ease colic, constipation, dyspepsia, flatulence and nausea.

When burned or vaporised it's used in cases of asthma and bronchitis and as an appetite suppressant for those with some eating disorders. It's also used to boost courage and mental strength.

Blends well with: You may find that Fennel blends particularly well with Lavender, Geranium, Sandalwood, Rose,

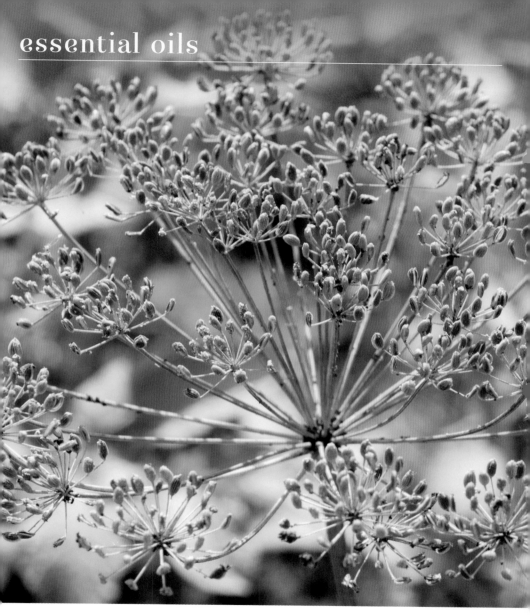

Bergamot, Black Pepper, Pine and the Citrus Oils.

Toxicity & safety: Always ensure you are using Sweet Fennel rather than Bitter Fennel. Sweet Fennel is non-irritant and relatively non-toxic. However, it may be narcotic in large doses and should be avoided altogether by epileptics, anyone with a kidney disorder and pregnant and nursing mothers.

frankincense

Boswellia carterii: *From the plant family Burseraceae.*

Originates from the area around the Red Sea, now also grown in Africa, particularly in the north-east in countries such as Somalia and Ethiopia.

Obtained by steam distillation of the resin of the tree.

Properties claimed for Frankincense essential oil include: Emmanagogue, expectorant, relaxing, rubefacient, sedative and tonic.

Summary: Frankincense is seen as a calming and balancing oil for the emotions and it's also used in remedies for the skin and lungs too.

History: The history of Frankincense goes back way before humans starting writing things down and it has long been one of the most popular plants used in natural remedies. In ancient times it was one of the most sought after and expensive substances and was highly valued for its ability to calm and assist in regulating the breathing. This made it very attractive to many different religions that still use it today in various ceremonies such as prayer and meditation.

The Ancient Egyptians and the Hebrews imported copious amounts from the Phoenicians. It was used for religious purposes and also as a perfume, in cosmetics and medicine. The Egyptians offered it to the gods while the Hebrews valued it extremely highly – according to the bible it was offered as a gift to the baby Jesus. For many centuries Frankincense was literally worth its weight in gold.

The trade in Frankincense had effects that still resonate today. The camel trains that delivered them soon grew to involve thousands of camels. Cities that still survive today were quickly established along the route and the well-trodden path through the Middle East towards the west can be seen from satellite images even today.

Nowadays Frankincense is found in soaps, cosmetics and perfumes as a fixative or a fragrance. Additionally it's used in some medicines such as throat pastilles and in tiny amounts in food and drink products.

Usage & methods of application: In massage Frankincense is often used in solutions aimed at improving respiratory conditions such as bronchitis and asthma. It's applied via a method of massage that concentrates on the chest and uses strokes to open up the chest. It's also commonly found in skincare creams and lotions.

Particularly suited to mature skin because of its tonic properties, Frankincense may

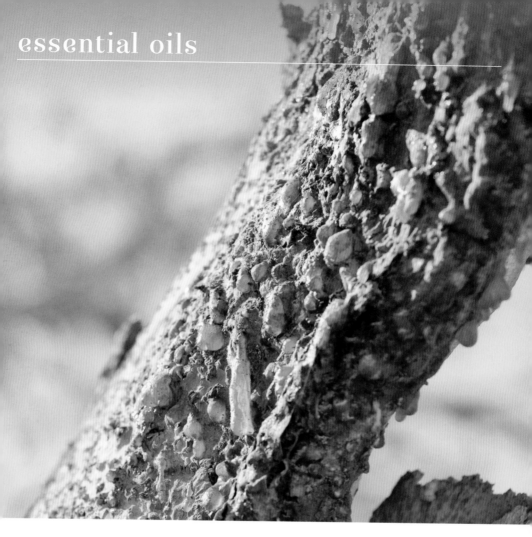

essential oils

help to tighten slack skin around the face and slow the appearance of wrinkles. It may even help to reduce wrinkles already present. When burned or vaporised Frankincense is again used to alleviate the symptoms of bronchial problems. It is also utilised as a calming oil which means it's often used during meditation as well as relieving anxiety (which again may be very useful for asthmatics in keeping them calm and avoiding the panic which can often worsen the condition).

Blends well with: Most essential oils blend well with one another. You may find that Frankincense blends especially well with Benzoin, Sandalwood, Lavender, Myrrh, Pine, Orange, Bergamot and Lemon.

Toxicity & safety: Frankincense is non-toxic and non-irritant and so can be used safely by the majority of people.

geranium

Pelargonium graveolens: From the plant family Geraniaceae.

Originally native to South Africa, now grown worldwide but especially in the Mediterranean, Russia, Europe and Egypt.

The oil is made from pretty much the whole plant – leaves, flowers and flower stalks.

Extracted by steam distillation.

Properties claimed for Geranium Essential Oil include: Astringent, antidepressant, diuretic, anti-inflammatory, balancing, haemostatic, vulnerary, vermifuge, stimulant, tonic and uplifting.

Summary: Geranium is another versatile oil with Aromatherapy benefits for both physical and mental ailments. It has a gorgeous and highly desirable aroma which also makes it hugely popular in the world of perfumery.

History: Geranium is another plant with a long history. It was used by the ancient Egyptians, predominantly for treating cancerous tumours. Early Africans are thought to have drunk tea made from the leaves of Geranium to cure stomach upsets and to stem internal bleeding.

Geranium plants and seeds were introduced to Europe via Holland in the sixteenth century and arrived in England in the early part of the seventeenth century when John Tradescant the Elder brought back some seeds after a trip to Paris. He was a royal gardener and a naturalist and was responsible for introducing Geranium to the UK.

Culpeper (early English authority on herbal medicine) described the use of Geranium in treating wounds in the seventeenth century and in the eighteenth century Geranium was used to treat haemorrhoids and swollen skin as well as being added to poultices to treat wounds and tumours.

In 1847 the French began to produce Geranium Oil from a territory island in the Indian Ocean. Victorians used Geranium to scent rooms, repel insects and in perfumes.

In modern times Geranium is often found in many commercially available products including soaps, shampoos, deodorants and perfumes.

Usage & methods of application: Commonly found in the treatment of skin conditions as it balances sebum production and helps to keep skin supple, tones dull skin. It's suitable for all skin types. It also improves circulation so can help to prevent chilblains, bruising

essential oils

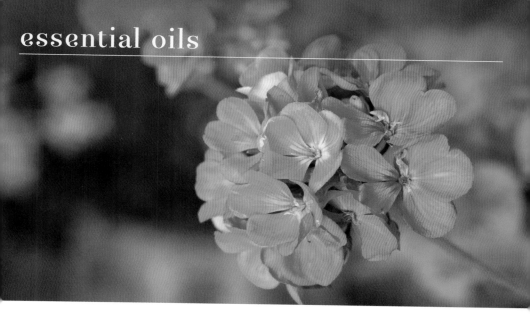

and broken capillaries. It's used to stimulate the lymphatic system and is a good oil to use in massage aimed at reducing the appearance of cellulite.

Mentally Geranium is regarded as a stimulant which can assist in lifting the spirits as well as relieving anxiety, stress and depression. The balancing properties of the oil mean that it is commonly used to alleviate the depressive symptoms of PMT, the menopause and heavy periods.

Geranium is a particularly lovely oil to burn or vaporise, as much for its beautiful aroma as for the potential mental and physical benefits. It does have decongestant properties and is an uplifting oil which can help to raise the spirits.

In massage Geranium is commonly used for clearing oily skin and moisturising dry skin and can help to lessen and prevent the appearance of scars and stretch marks. The balancing properties of the oil make it ideal to use in massage in

times of stress as it works both inside and outside the body – many women find using Geranium Oil in massage to alleviate the pain caused by PMT or the menopause to be hugely beneficial both physically and mentally.

The odour of insect repelling oils such as Citronella can be improved by blending with Geranium for a more floral and attractive aroma.

Blends well with: All essential oils generally blend well with one another. You may find that Geranium blends particularly well with Angelica, Basil, Bergamot, Carrot Seed, Cedarwood, Citronella, Clary Sage, Grapefruit, Jasmine, Lavender, Lime, Neroli, Orange and Rosemary.

Safety and toxicity: Geranium is regarded as a particularly safe oil but should not be used while pregnant or breastfeeding unless under the direct supervision of a qualified professional aromatherapist. People with very sensitive skin should avoid using Geranium.

ginger

Zingiber officinale: *From the plant family Zingiberaceae.*
Comes from India, China and tropical countries such as Jamaica, the West Indies and Nigeria.
The essential oil is produced by steam distillation of the root.
Properties claimed for Ginger essential oil include: Stimulating, tonic, analgesic, laxative, warming, rubefacient, antispasmodic and stomachic.

Summary: A wonderfully spicy and warming oil which is most often used for stimulating the circulation and enlivening tired bodies.

History: Ginger is an ancient remedy. The first documented use has been traced back to around 2000BC in China. It's still used in that country today to combat digestive upsets such as excessive flatulence and nausea, as do the Indian Ayurvedic people. Native Americans also documented use of the spice for these problems. It's also established a reputation as an aphrodisiac in several different cultures.

Confucious, Marco Polo and Dioscorides are some of the famous historical names who either wrote about Ginger or are known to have used it.

Ginger made its way to Europe in the Middle Ages via the Spice Route and was taken to South America by the Spaniards. Because it's such a lovely spice to use in flavouring food, it seems likely that the discovery of its perceived medical benefits were a happy accident after the positive effects of consuming the spice were noted. Prior to the 14th century Ginger was a very rare commodity

and was literally worth its weight in gold. People who became involved in the trade of Ginger were among the wealthiest around at the time. 1lb of Ginger was worth the equivalent of one sheep in the Middle Ages.

In modern times Ginger has been approved for use in Germany to alleviate nausea in pregnant women as well as to combat motion sickness.

Usage & methods of application:
As an oil Ginger is mainly used in massage albeit in a very low ratio and normally as part of a blend with other oils and a carrier oil. This is because it is a dermal irritant and so should always be used with care. It's used for treating tired and aching muscle and skeletal issues as well as general fatigue and also to help ease cramps caused by constipation or excessive flatulence.

You can burn or vaporise Ginger essential oil just like any other essential oil. Because it's a warming oil with good

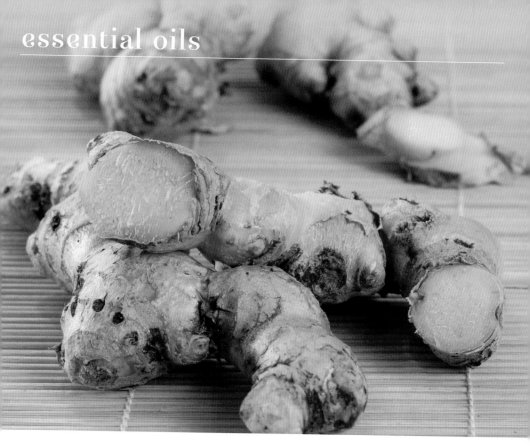

decongestant properties it's often burned to help unblock a stuffy nose. It's also used to liquefy and encourage the movement of sticky mucus and in the treatment of catarrhal lung conditions and chesty coughs.

In massage Ginger should always be very well diluted as it is an irritant to the skin in concentrations higher than around 1%. It's used in treating muscular pain, fatigue, rheumatism and arthritis. It stimulates circulation in the skin so is often used to help heal bruises and chilblains. You may find it simpler to just add a drop or two to an existing massage oil.

Blends well with: All essential oils generally blend well with one another. You may find that as Ginger has a particularly powerful aroma you'll need to use it in small concentrations so it doesn't overpower the other oils in your blend. Ginger blends particularly well with all citrus oils as well as Bergamot, Frankincense, Neroli, Rose, Sandalwood and Ylang Ylang.

Toxicity and safety: Ginger should be avoided altogether by those with sensitive skins and care should be taken by anyone planning to use it on the skin. It should always be very well diluted to a maximum of 1% in a carrier oil.

grapefruit

Citrus paradisi: From the plant family Rutaceae.

Comes from Tropical Asia, the West Indies, USA, Israel, Cuba among others.

Made from expression of the peel of the fruit.

Properties claimed for Grapefruit essential oil include: Astringent, depurative, diuretic, stimulant, tonic and uplifting.

Summary: As you might expect, Grapefruit is a refreshing oil with good uplifting properties. It's commonly used to counteract depression, fatigue and lethargy.

History: Grapefruit has a relatively short history compared to many essential oils. It wasn't until 1750 that the fruit was first described by the Welsh naturalist and author Griffith Hughes. He called it the "forbidden fruit of Barbados" which will give you some idea of where he discovered it. The fruit quickly became hugely popular and began to be cultivated in the West Indies and in warmer areas of North America.

The botanical origin of the fruit is something of a mystery. The best guess is that it's a hybrid fruit which was the result of a coming together of Shaddock (Citrus maxima) and the Sweet Orange (Citrus sinensis).

There is no record of deliberate hybridization to willingly produce the plant and searches of its native homelands have revealed no native growing trees so it's thought that Grapefruit is the result of a happy accident. This seems appropriate given the sunny and uplifting nature of the oil.

In modern times Grapefruit is used in a wide variety of soaps, cosmetics, perfumes and detergents as a fragrance. It's also found in many food and drink products.

Usage & methods of application: Primarily known for its wonderful uplifting properties, Grapefruit is a great oil to turn to in times of stress or depression. It's also used to alleviate fatigue and can stimulate immunity and so can be useful in warding off colds and flu.

Grapefruit is an astringent oil so is used to treat dull and oily skin as well as acne. It is often found in blends aimed at reducing cellulite and is a diuretic which can help to reduce water retention and oedema (dropsy).

Grapefruit is a beautiful oil to burn or vaporise. It can help to defend against airborne bugs and viruses and at the same time will infuse the air with its wonderfully uplifting aroma.

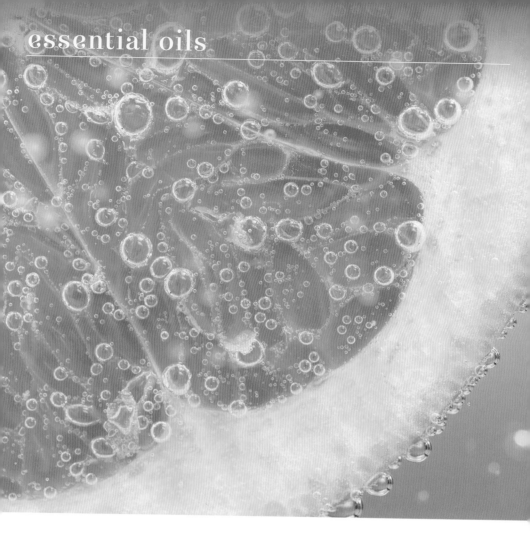

For use in massage or when blended in creams or lotions it should be diluted to 5% maximum. It's not a sensitising oil but care should still be taken. Unlike most citrus oils it's not a photosensitiser and can be used as a substitute for other citrus oils when photosensitivity is a problem.

Blends well with: All essential oils generally blend well with one another. You may find that Grapefruit blends particularly well with Bergamot, Lavender, Geranium, Palmarosa and Frankincense.

Toxicity and safety: Grapefruit is regarded as a safe oil and is not normally an irritant. It's best to look for Grapefruit oil which has been expressed rather than distilled as the latter version can cause problems in relation to phototoxicity. It's still advisable to dilute the expressed oil to a maximum of 5% before skin application.

juniperberry

Juniperus communis: From the plant family Cupressaceae.
Widely distributed in the Northern Hemisphere and also Africa and Central America.
The essential oil is obtained by steam distillation of the berries.
Properties claimed for Juniperberry essential oil include: Antiseptic, anti-rheumatic, antispasmodic, astringent, carminative, depurative, diuretic, rubefacient, stimulating, stomachic, sudorific, vulnerary and tonic.

Summary: Juniper is most used for its detoxifying properties which can have a positive effect on both the mind and body.

History: Juniper has long been used to prevent infection. Even until relatively recently sprigs of the plant were burned in French hospitals along with Rosemary to keep the atmosphere of hospital wards clean. There is also evidence of Juniper being used this way in many other countries from Tibet (where it is still revered today) to the UK. During the Black Death plague that swept through Europe it was one of the most popular ways to protect against the spread of the disease.

Juniper berries were also found in several ancient Egyptian tombs. There is no record of Juniper trees growing in Egypt so it's thought the berries probably came from Greece. The Greeks recorded the medicinal uses of Juniper berries well before they used it in foods and drinks.

Juniper is also thought to be a stimulant for the appetite and this may be a reason as to why Gin & Tonic has become such a popular aperitif.

Usage & methods of application: Juniper is an extremely versatile oil for which many applications have been established over the years.

In massage and skincare it is used to treat acne (especially where greasy skin is also a problem). Men especially prefer solutions made with juniper as it has a more masculine aroma than some of the other oils. It's often found in preparations aimed at detoxifying the body and used in small amounts it can also be helpful in combatting urine retention.

Massage blends including juniper are also used to combat adult colic, arthritis, cellulite, nervous tension, mild cystitis, liver problems, obesity and even hangovers.

When burned or vaporised, Juniper is commonly used to help with nervous tension, as a hangover reliever, after the overindulgence of food, to combat addictions and to uplift the

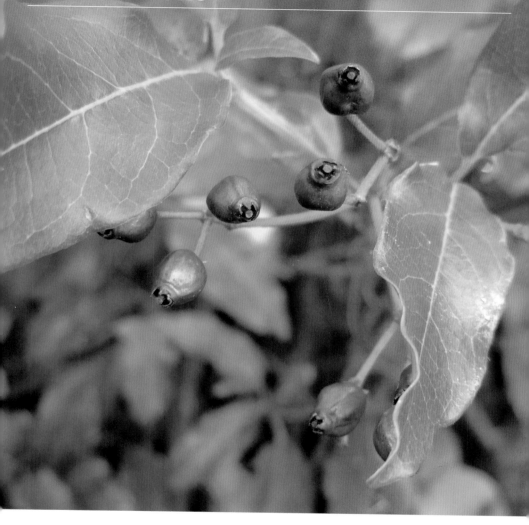

spirit during times of stress or when a boost in confidence is required.

Blends well with: Most essential oils blend well with one another. You may find that Juniperberry blends especially well with Cedarwood, Cypress, Geranium, Grapefruit, Lavender, Bergamot, Lime, Vetiver, Clary Sage and Lemongrass.

Toxicity & safety: Generally considered to be a non-toxic oil, Juniperberry should still be avoided by pregnant and nursing mothers or by those with kidney problems as it has the potential to stimulate the uterine muscles. Prolonged misuse may cause damage to the kidneys.

lavender

Lavendula Angustifolia: From the plant family Lamiaceae (Labiatae)
Originates from Mediterranean countries and all over Europe including England.
The oil is made from the flower of the plant.
Extracted by steam distillation.
Properties: Analgesic, anti-inflammatory, antiseptic, antispasmodic,
antiviral, balancing, cooling, detoxifying, fungicidal, hypotensive, relaxing,
sedative and tonic.

Summary: Perhaps the most well-known of all essential oils, Lavender is a staple oil for anyone practising Aromatherapy and is also a great oil to keep at home for minor scratches, to aid relaxation and because of its gorgeous aroma.

The safest of the oils, Lavender is a great oil to start off your collection because of its versatility and the fact that it's comparatively low in cost.

Anyone who has experienced the sensation of walking through a beautiful, vibrant field of lavender in full bloom will recognise the evocative scent from this beautiful oil.

History: Lavender has been used throughout the ages for both its medicinal strengths and for its wonderful aroma as a perfume. It has become associated in many cultures with cleanliness, love and healing.

The ancient Greeks used Lavender to combat chest pains, constipation and throat infections. Romans used it in their baths, for cooking and simply for scenting the air (things could get a bit smelly at that time!).

Medieval and renaissance Europeans used Lavender as a disinfectant and a deodorant. They scattered the plant on the stone floors of castles and homes.

During London's Great Plague in the 17th century, Lavender was in great demand. People wore bunches tied to their wrists to ward off infection and thieves who were robbing the graves and homes of Plague sufferers concocted a mixture containing Lavender known as "Four Thieves Vinegar" to protect themselves.

This might all seem a bit naive but we now know that the plague was spread by fleas. We also know that Lavender repels these insects so the positive effect of wearing Lavender in these times should not be underestimated!

essential oils

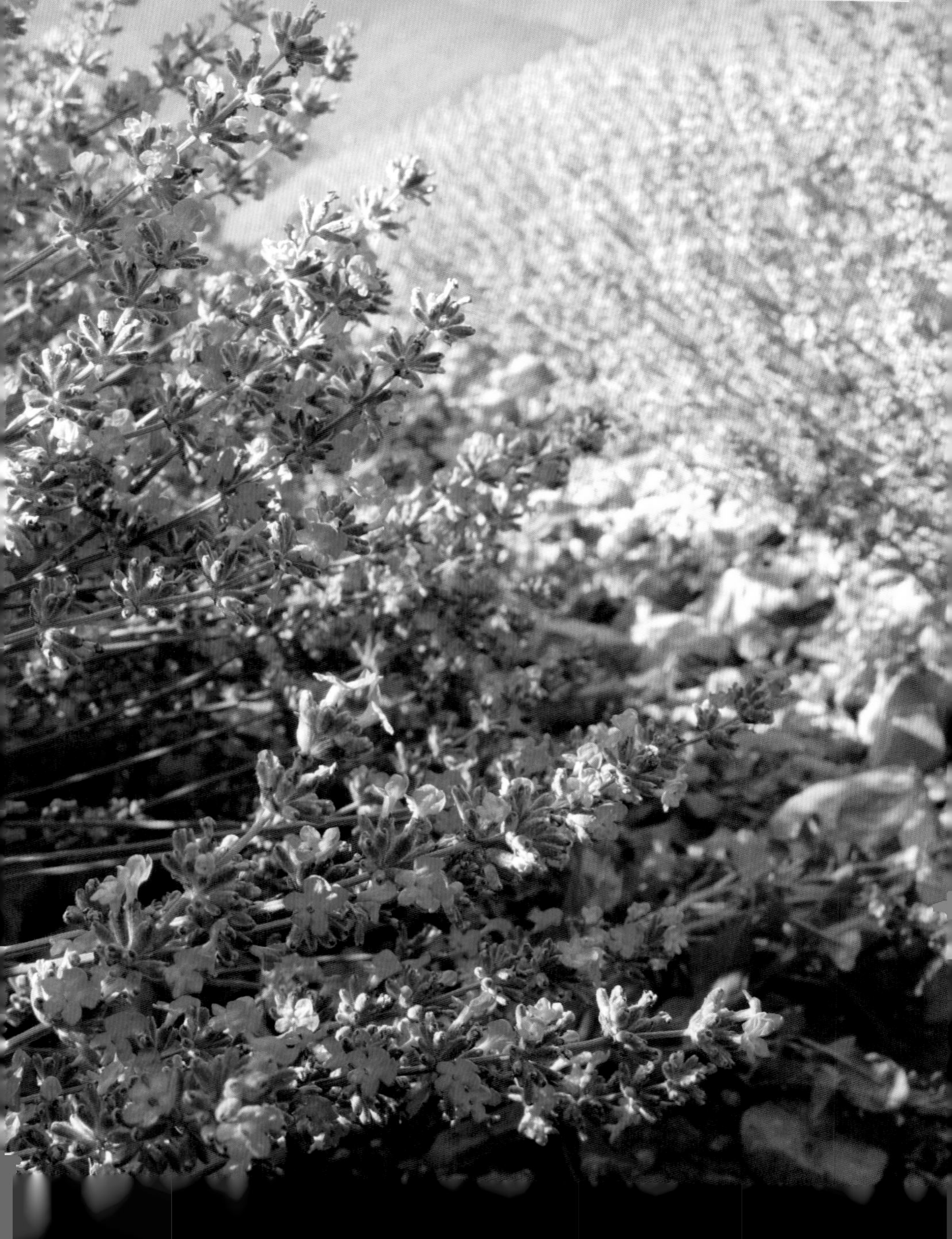

Modern day aromatherapists use Lavender to treat many different physical symptoms. It's excellent for treating burns and will help the skin to recover quickly as well as lessening the appearance of any scarring. These same properties also make it great for soothing sunburn.

It can also balance the production of sebum in oily skin and is a soothing antiseptic for insect bites and stings. It can be very helpful in cases of dermatitis. It's also thought to help lower high blood pressure and is a calming oil that is great for stress-related conditions such as palpitations.

Lavender can ease bronchitis, laryngitis and relax laboured breathing. It's also antiviral and so can help to ward off flu and colds.

Lavender can also sooth and relieve muscular aches, strains and pains through massage application as well as soothing the problems caused by rheumatism.

One advantage of introducing essential oils to your routine is not only the physical benefits but the mental boosts they can also offer. Lavender is perhaps the greatest example of this holistic approach as it's a wonderfully calming oil.

It can help to balance the emotions and may be especially useful during times of depression. It's a stress relieving oil which can help reduce insomnia, anxiety and tension. Also good to sniff or burn after a shock as well as being beneficial to those suffering from headaches or migraines.

There have been some interesting studies carried out in the effects of Lavender over the years.

One study showed that workers who sniffed Lavender at the beginning of their lunch breaks returned to work with more energy than a control group who hadn't inhaled any Lavender. The study suggested that because the group that had sniffed Lavender had been able to relax more deeply during their lunch hour they were less likely to suffer the post lunch slump that affects so many people.

Further studies show that massage with Lavender Oil can be hugely beneficial to those suffering from sleep disorders such as insomnia. Results showed improved sleep, a more stable mood and increased brain capacity the next day as well as reduction in anxiety.

It also appears that Lavender may be useful in controlling post-operative pain. A group of patients were given oxygen infused with Lavender and reported higher satisfaction with the pain relief provided compared to another group who were given just plain oxygen.

In Germany Lavender flowers in tea have been approved as a suitable treatment for insomnia, restlessness and stomach complications caused by nervous conditions.

Lavender is one of the oldest known ingredients in perfumery and is used extensively by big name brands in skincare, hair care and beauty creams and products. It's also found in some foods and drinks.

Usage & methods of application:
It's effective when burned or vaporised. Physically it can help in relieving stress, can fight airborne bacteria and viruses and

may also assist in relieving headaches and migraines. It can alleviate laboured breathing and may ease the symptoms of bronchitis and laryngitis. Mentally it's one of the oils most commonly used in stress relief, to calm and balance the emotions and to relax.

When used in massage Lavender Oil can promote cell growth and rapid healing for scars, stretch marks and burns as well as balancing sebum production to combat greasy or oily skin. It is an antiseptic so great for gently soothing insect bites, stings and minor wounds and is also good for people suffering with dermatitis.

When used neat (see safety advice below), Lavender can fight bacterial

infections such as Athlete's Foot and cold sores. It can help to prevent infection in blisters as well as soothe them.

Blends well with: Most essential oils generally blend well with one another. You may find that Lavender blends particularly well with Cedarwood, Clary Sage, Geranium, Pine, Nutmeg and all the citrus oils.

Toxicity & safety: Lavender is probably the safest of all the essential oils. It may cause sensitisation in a tiny minority of people. If you develop any sort of reaction then you should stop using the oil immediately. It's generally thought that Lavender is safe for use by pregnant women but conclusive research has yet to be undertaken so it's a decision for the individual.

There are some indications that Lavender may affect the hormonal balance of boys who are yet to reach puberty and so it should be used sparingly with this particular age group. There are no contraindications for girls of the same age.

It can be applied neat to minor skin abrasions and wounds but great care should always be taken. If you are unsure about using it neat please seek the advice of a qualified aromatherapist.

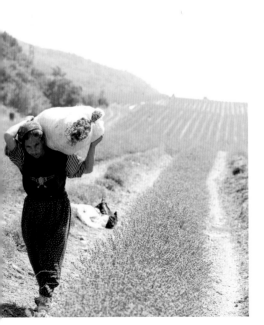

lemon

Citrus limon: *From the plant family Rutaceae*

Lemon trees are found and cultivated the world over. Originally native to Asia and India, they also grow wild in Mediterranean countries including Spain and Italy.

The essential oil is cold pressed from the peel of the fruit.

Properties claimed for Lemon essential oil include: Antiseptic, antiviral, detoxifying, depurative, diuretic, fungicidal, haemostatic, hypotensive, stimulant, tonic and uplifting.

Summary: Lemon is known as a protecting and stimulating oil which is used to aid the body's natural defensive systems and lift the spirits and emotions.

History: Lemon is a fruit which has stirred strong emotions throughout its history. The origins of the fruit trees are not known but it's thought likely that they first grew in and around India or Southeast Asia before spreading to China where it is known that Lemon trees have been cultivated for at least 4000 years. It eventually made its way to the Arab world before coming to the attention of the Roman Empire.

The Crusaders were almost certainly responsible for introducing Lemon to Europe and by the Middle Ages it was known to the English. The true health giving value of the fruit was not realised until the great sea voyages in the 1500s when it was discovered that Lemon was the perfect solution to the huge problem of scurvy.

Lemon trees became so popular amongst the higher echelons of society during the renaissance that it became extremely fashionable to grow the trees much further north than their natural habitat. This lead to the construction of special conservatories to enable the trees to survive.

It was Columbus who was responsible for introducing Lemon to the New World – he took some seeds with him on one of his fantastic journeys and planted them in Hispaniola.

Usage & methods of application: A refreshing and uplifting oil, Lemon is often used in blends for burning or vaporising to stimulate the mind and encourage clarity of thought. Its antiseptic properties also mean it's used to protect against colds and flu. It's also thought to stimulate the immune system.

It is included in massage blends (in low concentrations) for the skin where it can be useful for treating boils, warts and acne. It can also benefit the circulatory

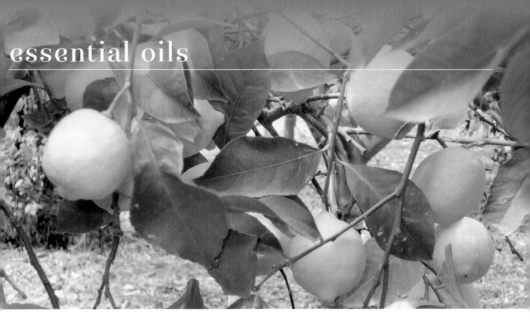

system, varicose veins and may help to lower overly high blood pressure.

Lemon is commonly found in many commercially available creams, lotions, perfumes, toothpastes and ointments.

In massage it should always be diluted to no more than 5% before skin application. Lemon is another oil that is good to add to your existing skincare or beauty products. Start with 1 drop, mix well and add more if you feel necessary.

In common with many citrus and other essential oils Lemon is a great oil to use around the house too. Try adding 10-15 drops to a spray bottle filled with water along with a couple of drops of natural soap for a great general purpose household cleaner. Alternatively add 4 drops Lemon and Lavender, 3 drops of Eucalyptus and a couple drops of Rosemary to a spray bottle filled with water. Shake well before each use and you will find this makes a great, natural cleaner for tops and surfaces.

Always perform a patch test on an out of sight corner to ensure the surface you're cleaning will not be adversely affected by the oils (you should do this with commercially available cleaners too).

Another household use for Lemon is as a natural stain remover on clothes and furniture. Simply add a drop or two to the affected area, allow to rest for a while then wash as normal. Always check that the material you are using the oil on is suitable by dabbing a small amount on an unobtrusive corner of the item in question.

Blends well with: All essential oils generally blend well with one another. You may find that Lemon blends particularly well with Lavender, Rose, Sandalwood, Benzoin, Eucalyptus, Geranium, Fennel, Juniper and Neroli.

Toxicity & safety: Lemon is a phototoxic oil so should not be used before or during a spell in the sun. It can cause skin irritation so should always be well diluted in a carrier oil or lotion when applied via massage.

lemongrass

Cymbopogon citratus: *From the plant family Poaceae.*
Grows in Asia, the West Indies and East India.
The essential oil is obtained by steam distillation of the dried grass.
Properties claimed for Lemongrass include: Antidepressant, antiseptic, astringent, stimulant, tonic and uplifting.

Summary: A wonderfully refreshing and stimulating oil for muscles, skin and the soul.

History: Lemongrass has only relatively recently pricked the consciousness of westerners thanks to the spread of Asian cuisine to the rest of the world. However, the herb and the oil have a long history of use in Asia stretching back over thousands of years. The Chinese use Lemongrass to treat a range of ailments including stomach pain, rheumatism, headaches and colds.

It's long been used in traditional Indian medicine, most often in the treatment of infectious diseases and fevers due to its powerful antiseptic and bactericidal properties.

The Ancient Greeks, Romans and Egyptians are also known to have used Lemongrass as an ingredient in cosmetics and perfumes.

In modern times Lemongrass is commonly found as a fragrance in soaps, cosmetics, perfumes and cleaning products. It's also used as a flavouring ingredient in many foods and drinks.

Usage & methods of application: Lemongrass has many potential uses in Aromatherapy. In skincare it's often blended with a base lotion or cream and used to treat oily skin, acne, for toning open pores and in insect repellent lotions.

In massage Lemongrass is commonly found in preparations to soothe aching joints and muscles as well as toning muscles, easing tired legs and fatigued bodies. It's often found in sport massage blends. It can be used to stimulate the appetite and relieve indigestion through massage too.

When burned or vaporised it is used to stimulate, revive and energise the emotions and relieve stress related conditions as well as easing nervous exhaustion. It's an antiseptic and is used to help avoid infections, sore throats and laryngitis and reduce fevers.

Blends well with: Most essential oils blend well with one another. You may find that Lemongrass blends especially well with Basil, Cedarwood, Coriander, Geranium, Jasmine, Lavender and Tea Tree.

Toxicity & safety: Lemongrass is generally regarded as non-toxic but may irritate sensitive skin if used improperly.

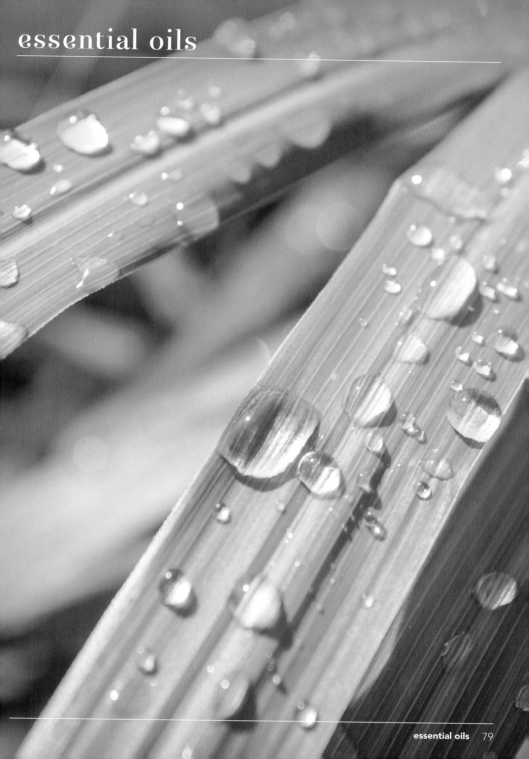

essential oils

lime

Citrus aurantifolia: *From the plant family Rutaceae.*

Thought to be native to south Asia but now found in many tropical and subtropical regions around the globe. Mainly cultivated in Mexico, Florida, the West Indies and Italy.

The oil is obtained by distillation of the Lime fruit.

Properties claimed for Lime essential oil include: Antiseptic, antiviral, aperitif, bactericidal, febrifuge, restorative and tonic.

Summary: Lime is regarded as an uplifting and revitalising oil with additional benefits to the immune system.

History: The most famous historical use of Lime is probably in the fight against scurvy amongst sailors in the 19th century. British sailors in particular benefited from a daily allowance of citrus fruits – initially Lemon with Lime being introduced later on. The high Vitamin C content was extremely valuable and Limes were easy to source as the British Navy sailed around the West Indies.

The use of citrus fruits like this became a closely guarded military secret and enabled the British to stay at sea for much longer periods than the navies of their enemies at the time. This is how British sailors became known as "Limeys".

The history of Lime stretches back a few centuries before this. It's thought it was introduced to eastern Mediterranean countries and Africa by the Arabs around 1000AD. It found its way to western Mediterranean countries in the 12th or 13th centuries via the Crusaders and Columbus is thought to have taken Lime seeds on his second voyage in 1493 leading to trees appearing in the West Indies, Mexico and Florida in the years following.

Nowadays Lime can be found in soaps, detergents, cosmetics and perfumes as well as in drinks and other foods. It's found in the world's most popular cola drink. The juice is used to produce Citric Acid.

Usage & methods of application: Lime and Lemon essential oils are pretty much interchangeable so it mostly depends on which aroma you prefer. When blended for massage, Lime is used in treatments for arthritis, cellulitis, high blood pressure, poor circulation and rheumatism. It's used to help with achy muscles and joints and cellulite. It is also blended in a lotion or cream when it can be helpful in clearing oily and congested skin and again to lessen the appearance of cellulite.

essential oils

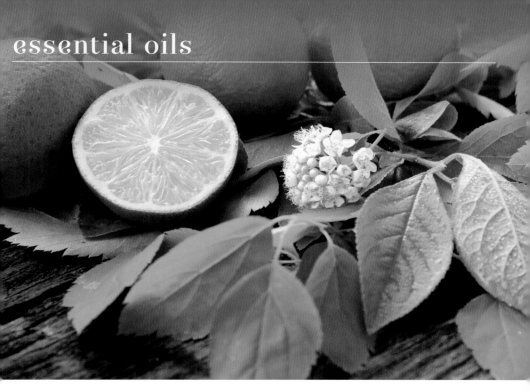

Lime is burned or vaporised to help with respiratory problems such as those associated with a cold, asthma or other bronchial issues. It's also regarded as an uplifting oil which is good to use in times of anxiety, stress or depression. Its antiseptic properties also mean that it's often burned to ward off infection and viruses and as a preventative measure during any illnesses of this type.

Lime is another oil which is very well suited to being used around the house. You can add it to your existing household cleaning products or come up with your own mixture. It works well on its own when added to clean water in a spray bottle to be used as a general cleaner for tops and surfaces. Alternatively you can add 10-15 drops to filtered water in a bottle with a fine spray attachment and use it as an air freshener.

There are lots of other ideas for using essential oils as a replacement for the chemical packed commercially available cleaning products available on the high street which you can find via a quick search on the internet.

Blends well with: Most essential oils generally blend well with one another. You may find that Lime blends especially well with Neroli, Lavender, Clary Sage and Ylang Ylang as well as the other citrus oils.

Toxicity & safety: Lime is a non-toxic oil but may cause irritation or sensitisation to the skin in some individuals if misused. It is phototoxic so should not be used on the skin before or during a spell in the sun.

mandarin

Citrus nobilis: *From the plant family Rutaceae.*

Native to southern China and the Far East. Now found worldwide and produced mainly in Italy, Spain, Algeria, Cyprus, Greece, the Middle East, Argentina and Brazil.

The oil is obtained by expression from the peel of the fruit.

Properties claimed for Mandarin essential oil include: Antiseptic, antispasmodic, carminative, digestive, diuretic and laxative (both mild), sedative, stimulant and tonic.

Summary: A refreshing oil with a happy character that is great for the whole family.

History: Ancient texts show that the fruit has been cultivated in China since 1100BC. They have long been regarded as a very special fruit. For many years they were exclusively reserved for use by the King and later they became a gift for honoured statesmen. It's still revered in China but is now available to the mass population who regard the mandarin as a symbol of good fortune and prosperity and consume the fruit as part of the Chinese New Year celebrations.

Mandarins didn't reach Europe until the early 19th century. The Natural Historian Sir Abraham Hume brought back two plants to England from a trip to China. It eventually spread throughout Europe and the rest of the world. Mandarin is commonly known as Tangerine in the USA.

Nowadays Mandarin can be found in soaps, perfumes, cosmetics and colognes. It's also used as a flavouring agent in sweets, drinks and liqueurs.

Usage & methods of application: In massage Mandarin is often used in blends to treat digestive problems, dyspepsia and other intestinal issues. It's also used to treat cellulitis, stretch marks and fluid retention. It can be found in skincare blends aimed at relieving acne, congested and oily skin, spots and acts as a general tonic to the skin.

When burned or vaporised Mandarin is regarded as a "happy" oil and can evoke feelings of joy and uplifted emotions. It's a good oil to burn around children as it has a gentle action and is used to promote sleep, calm restlessness and nervous tension. It's often burned as part of a synergistic blend with other citrus oils.

Blends well with: Most essential oils blend well with one another. You may find that Mandarin blends especially well with all citrus oils as well as Cinnamon, Clary Sage, Clove, Frankincense, Lavender and Nutmeg.

essential oils

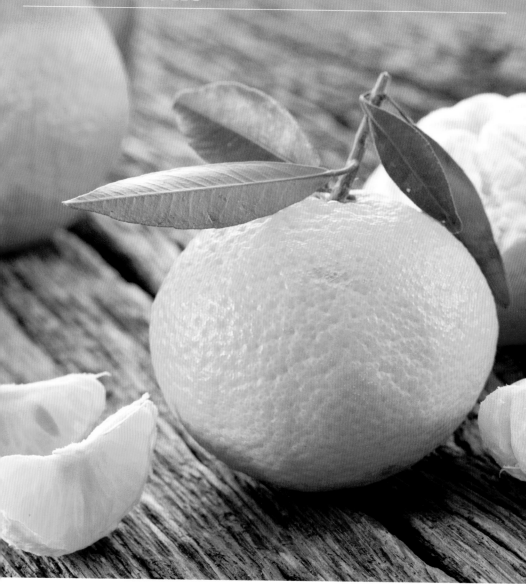

Toxicity & safety: Non-toxic, non-sensitising and non-irritant, Mandarin is one of very few oils that are safe to use after the first trimester of pregnancy. It's possibly phototoxic so shouldn't be used on the skin before or during a spell in the sun.

marjoram

Origanum majorana: From the plant family Lamiaceae (Labiatae).
Grows principally in Mediterranean countries such as Egypt, France and Spain as well as parts of North Africa.
The oil is obtained by steam distillation of the leaves of the plant.
Properties claimed for Marjoram include: Analgesic, antispasmodic, emmenagogue, relaxing, sedative, tonic, nervine, laxative, vulnerary, vasodilatory, warming and hypotensive.

Summary: Soothing and comforting, great for calming a busy brain. A warming and clearing oil which can be of great comfort in times of anxiety or distress. It's also considered to be one of the best oils to use in the treatment of bronchial problems such as asthma.

History: Named "The herb of happiness" by the Romans, Marjoram has been used for centuries in traditional folk medicine. The Ancient Greeks used it in their medicines, fragrances and cosmetics – the Latin name Origanum derives from a Greek word meaning "joy of the mountains". The Ancient Egyptians used it for its healing properties and also to help with grief.

It was common in many 17th century English gardens and escaped to grow wild too. Nicholas Culpeper noted that it was helpful for "all diseases of the chest" and that it encouraged easier breathing.

Usage & methods of application: Marjoram is most commonly used in Aromatherapy for its warming properties. In massage it gives a feeling of warmth as it dilates the capillaries just under the skin. This makes it a common ingredient in massage blends for loosening tight and painful muscles especially after tough physical activity. It's also used to reduce the pain of arthritis and rheumatism as the warming effect can often enable joints that have stiffened up to loosen again and so enable gentle exercise etc.

When burned, vaporised or used in a steam inhalation Marjoram is often recommended for helping to clear a congested chest. It's regarded as especially effective in cases of asthma, bronchitis and colds.

A hot bath with a few drops of Marjoram can be very beneficial to those suffering a heavy cold. It's even thought to help with a tickly cough when gently massaged around the throat and neck.

Burning or vaporising the oil is also a good way to calm a busy mind, soothe and relax those with high tension or hyperactivity

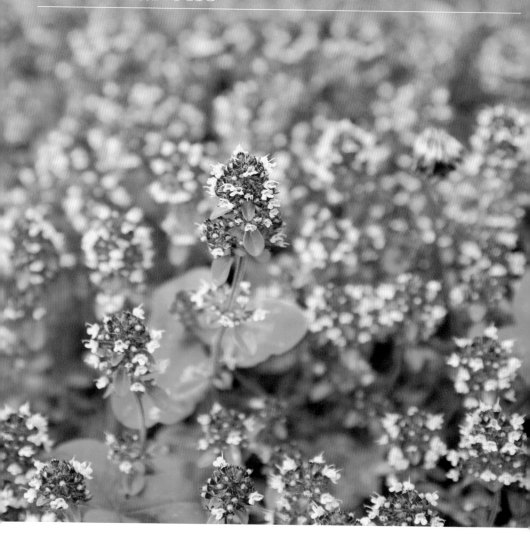

and generally bring about a feeling of well-being and happiness. People who are lonely or grief-stricken will often have Marjoram recommended to them.

Blends well with: Most essential oils blend well with one another. You may find that Marjoram blends especially well with Lavender, Cypress, Cedarwood, Chamomile, Bergamot, Eucalyptus and Tea Tree.

Toxicity & safety: Marjoram is an emmenagogue and should be strictly avoided during pregnancy. Otherwise it's a safe oil which is non-toxic, non-sensitising and non-irritant if used correctly.

orange

Citrus aurantium dulcis: *From the family Rutaceae.*

Bred first by orange-growers in China, the sweet orange is now widely cultivated in subtropical regions, especially Brazil, the USA, China and India.

The oil comes from the thick peel and rind of the orange fruit.

Method of extraction is cold expression.

Properties claimed for Orange Essential Oil include: Antidepressant, anti-inflammatory, antiseptic, bactericidal, carminative, choleretic, digestive, fungicidal, hyposensitive, sedative (nervous), stimulant, (digestive and lymphatic), stomachic and tonic.

Summary: Sweet orange is the world's most popular fruit, rich in vitamins A, B, and C. The essential oil is widely available and produced in such high quantities that it's normally a very inexpensive oil. It's considered to be a versatile palliative to many ailments.

History: Oranges have been grown in East Asia for as long as human civilisation has been recorded. While the original plant is thought to originate from India and Indochina, the sweet orange was cultivated in China due to the demand for a larger, sweeter fruit by the Imperial nobility. The orange, rich in vitamins, became a staple of Chinese traditional medicine. According to the famed Ming-Dynasty herbalist, Li Shizhen, "The fruits of all the different species and varieties of citrus are considered by the Chinese to be cooling... the sweet varieties increase bronchial secretion, and the sour promote expectoration. They all quench thirst, and are stomachic and carminative."

The first appearance of oranges in Europe was in the markets of the Roman Empire. These first imports were due to the efforts of Persian traders, but it was not until the 16th Century that the sweet variety was brought to the Mediterranean by the Portuguese. The sweet orange is often called the "Portuguese orange" in Southern Europe as a result.

The popularity of the orange in Europe led to its cultivation in the Americas by Spanish colonists, with the first plantation believed to have begun on the island of Cananeia, off Sao Paulo, in the mid 16th century. Oranges have since been grown worldwide, being largely produced in Brazil and the USA as well as remaining popular in their countries of origin, India and China.

Usage & methods of application: Orange is a highly versatile oil with a range of applications. Chinese traditional medicine traditionally uses orange peel

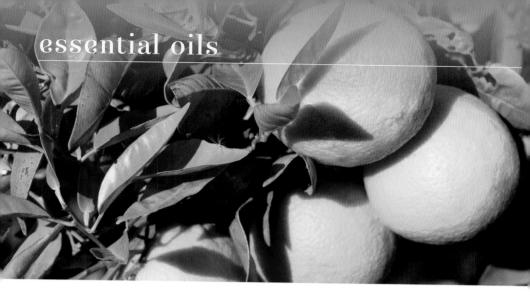

(from which the oil is expressed) to treat coughs, colds, and anorexia.

It is anti-inflammatory and thought to provide quick relief for mild irritation or pain. It's also used as an antispasmodic as it relaxes the mental and muscular systems. Its antiseptic properties inhibit the growth of microbes and bacteria, so it can be used to aid the disinfection of wounds.

Orange oil is also used to relax the digestive system so is commonly used as a carminative and diuretic as well as to target indigestion. It's often found in blends to reduce menstrual cramps, for aiding the expulsion of digestive gases and to relieve constipation.

Orange oil, when used as part of a face wash, is often used to rejuvenate and tone the skin. Additionally, its cheerful, fresh and fruity aroma may help to reduce stress and anxiety.

Orange is an excellent oil to burn or vaporise as its fresh and fruity aroma will quickly clear the air in a stuffy or musty room. Citrus fruits are cooling, calming scents and orange is the sweetest of these.

It's often used in blends to assist relaxation of both mind and muscles, as well as blends aimed at assisting the improvement of circulation and reducing cramps, aches or pains.

Orange oil can also be added to a body wash, lotion or liquid soap to help to moisturise the skin as well. Start with a couple of drops and increase the amount as you feel necessary.

Blends well with: Most essential oils generally blend well with one another. You may find that orange blends particularly well with Lavender, Neroli, Clary Sage, Myrrh, Nutmeg, Cinnamon and Clove.

Toxicity & safety: Orange is generally a safe oil. Limonene, in which Orange is rich, can be an irritant to some types of skin.

patchouli

Pogostemon cablin: *From the plant family Rutaceae.*

Originally from tropical Asia, mostly Indonesia and the Philippines. Still cultivated in these countries as well as India, China, Malaysia and South America.

The essential oil is obtained by steam distillation of the dried and fermented leaves of the plant.

Properties claimed for Patchouli essential oil include: Antidepressant, anti-inflammatory, antimicrobial, antiphlogistic, antiseptic, antitoxic, antiviral, aphrodisiac, astringent, bactericidal, carminative, deodorant, digestive, diuretic, febrifuge, fungicidal, prophylactic, nervous stimulant, stomachic and tonic.

Summary: Patchouli is one of those oils that people love or hate. It has a persistent, lingering aroma and often only a small amount is needed in a blend for positive results. It's an uplifting oil that also has sedative properties.

History: A divisive oil which rocketed to prominence during the 1960s and the rise of the Flower Power movement. No specific reasons are known as to why Patchouli suddenly became so popular but it's possible that the heavy, penetrating odour gave those wearing it a feeling of mysticism and perhaps even put them in mind of India. Or maybe it was worn for its deodorising properties, its reputation as an aphrodisiac or for its capacity to cover some of the other "exotic" smells common at the time.

Before then it's thought that leaves of Patchouli were used by Chinese traders travelling to the Middle East to protect silk cloth from egg laying moths. It's thought that this led to Patchouli becoming popular with Europeans at the time – it's even said that Queen Victoria's linen chests were protected by Patchouli.

The Chinese, Japanese and Malaysians use the herb to treat colds, nausea, headaches, vomiting and halitosis while the latter two countries also use it as an antidote to snake bites.

Today Patchouli is commonly found as a fixative in perfumes and soaps and is used in foods and drinks as a flavouring agent. It's used as a masking agent to disguise nasty smells and tastes.

Usage & methods of application: Patchouli is fairly unusual among essential oils in that it improves with age. It should be used in small amounts. In Aromatherapy massage blends it's used on scars, chapped skin and to encourage cell growth. It's also used to relieve stress and related conditions, anxiety and to stimulate the digestive system.

essential oils

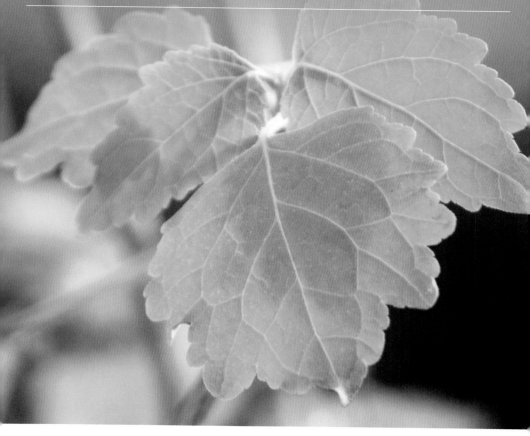

In a cream or lotion Patchouli is often used against fungal infections such as athlete's foot. It's also used to fight skin infections, regenerate the skin, speed up healing while lessening the chances of unattractive scars appearing and also to treat acne, eczema, ulcers and scalp disorders.

When burned or vaporised Patchouli is regarded as a good stress reliever and is used to relieve lethargy and anxiety. You may also find that it helps to create a romantic atmosphere and is also a good insect repellent.

Blends well with: Most essential oils blend well with one another. You may find that Patchouli blends especially well with Bergamot, Clary Sage, Geranium, Lavender and Myrrh.

Toxicity & safety: Patchouli can cause phototoxicity so should not be used before or during a spell in the sun. Otherwise it's non-toxic, non-sensitising and non-irritant. Some people just can't stand the aroma of Patchouli and may feel nauseous when they smell it. It may also cause a loss of appetite in some people if used in too large amounts.

peppermint

Mentha arvensis: *From the plant family Lamiaceae (Labiatae).*

Peppermint grows worldwide but major producers are the USA, India and China. It's native to Southern Europe.

The essential oil is produced by steam distillation of the flowering herb and leaves.

Properties claimed for Peppermint essential oil include: Analgesic, antiseptic, antispasmodic, antiviral, antipruritic, carminative, cephalic, cooling, digestive tonic, expectorant, febrifuge, stimulant, stomachic, vermifuge, uplifting and vasoconstrictive.

Summary: Peppermint, as you'd expect, is regarded as a cooling and refreshing oil with many varied applications. It's also used via massage as a digestive aid.

History: Evidence shows that Peppermint is another plant that has been used for medicinal purposes for thousands of years. Traces of Peppermint have been found in Egyptian tombs dating back to 1000BC. Ancient Chinese and Japanese peoples also harvested the plant for medicinal and food use.

The Romans used Peppermint for similar purposes and also wore garlands of the herb while attending the great Roman feasts. During the 18th and 19th century England was one of the biggest producers of Peppermint. Eastern and Western cultures used Peppermint extensively for several different ailments. It was introduced to North America in the 19th century.

Usage & methods of application:
In Aromatherapy Peppermint has several uses. Perhaps the most appreciated is in its use to treat the nervous system. When burned or vaporised it's an oil

that may help to waken and freshen the mind, improve concentration, lessen mental fatigue, combat headaches and depression as well as calming anger or hysteria. It's also a decongestant which many people find very useful for unblocking sinuses and cold and flu symptoms as well as easing the symptoms of asthma and bronchial congestions.

When applied to the skin it's used as a cooling and refreshing oil – you'll often find it in Fresh Feet blends for example. These blends make use of its deodorising effect and also may soothe aching feet. It's commonly used in cooling creams to calm rashes and hives and can also be found in blends aimed at reducing pain and fever.

Commercially Peppermint is found in many consumables including toothpastes, cough and cold remedies, perfumes and household cleaning products.

essential oils

Peppermint is a very popular oil for use in burners and vaporisers. It can overpower other oils so caution should be applied when used in blends for burning. When used in this way it's commonly found in blends aimed at refreshing a room, clearing nasty odours, increasing concentration and stimulating the mind. It's also used as an insect repellent and to clear headaches and feelings of nausea.

In skincare and massage Peppermint should be diluted to 5% or less in a carrier oil. It's a very refreshing and enlivening oil so best avoided during the evening or at bed time.

Blends well with: All essential oils generally blend well with one another. You may find that Peppermint blends particularly well with Benzoin, Eucalyptus, Lavender, Marjoram, Lemon and Rosemary.

Toxicity & safety: Peppermint is thought to have a negative effect on homeopathic remedies and should not be used with or stored near them. It should not be used by people with heart disease or epilepsy. You should also avoid using Peppermint in the evening or when trying to relax and switch off – it's just too lively!

rose geranium

Pelargonium graveolens: *From the plant family Geraniaceae.*

Originally found in South Africa, Madagascar, Egypt and Morocco before being introduced to European countries such as Italy and Spain in the 17th Century.

The essential oil is obtained by steam distillation of the flowers, leaves and stalks of the plant.

Properties claimed for Rose Geranium essential oil include: Antidepressant, antiseptic, astringent, diuretic, deodorant, haemostatic, tonic and vulnerary.

Summary: One of the most uplifting of oils, Rose Geranium is a lovely oil to burn or vaporise due to its ability to impart positive feelings and its gorgeous aroma. It's also commonly found in skincare preparations due to the astringent nature of the oil and again for the wonderful fragrance. Rose Geranium is a different oil from both Rose and Geranium and should not be confused with the two.

History: Rose Geranium does not have the history behind it that a lot of essential oils have and didn't make it to Europe until the 17th century. Before that it's believed that it was used in its native Africa to treat burns and problems with the skin such as acne or boils.

It's also thought that it was initially utilised in the West as a houseplant which was used to ward off evil spirits. However, this is just as likely to have been because it smelt nice and helped to disguise the rather pungent smells common in homes at the time!

In modern times Rose Geranium is used extensively in perfumery, toothpastes, mouthwashes and as a flavouring in many foods and drinks.

Usage & methods of application: Rose Geranium is an extremely versatile oil which is used in many different ways in Aromatherapy. In massage it's used in blends for all skin types thanks to its astringent properties. A balancing oil which is used to regulate both oily and dry skins, it's also a cleansing oil which means it's often used for congested skin.

Amongst other things Rose Geranium is commonly found in massage treatments aimed at helping to alleviate the symptoms of PMS, depression, stress, anxiety, tension, fluid retention, eczema, shingles, cellulite, bruises, haemorrhoids and menstrual irregularities.

Like many essential oils Rose Geranium is a lovely oil to use in the bath for the same reasons it's used in massage – as well as

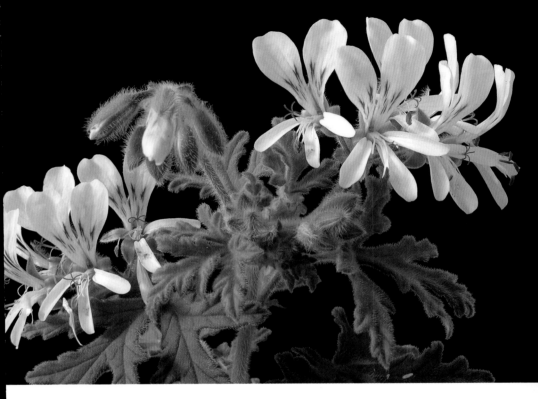

its lovely aroma. Simply add a couple of drops to a tablespoon of milk to help it disperse in the water.

When burned or vaporised Rose Geranium is again used to relieve stress, depression, anxiety and tension. It's soothing and calming so can also be used to alleviate PMS, menopausal problems and its energising properties mean it's often used to relieve excessive tiredness.

Blends well with: Essential oils generally blend well with one another. You may find that Rose Geranium blends particularly well with Angelica, Basil, Bergamot, Carrot Seed, Cedarwood, Citronella, Clary Sage, Grapefruit, Jasmine, Lavender, Lime, Neroli, Orange and Rosemary.

Toxicity & safety: Non-toxic, non-irritant and non-sensitising, Rose Geranium is generally considered to be a safe oil to use. It's probably best to avoid during pregnancy and if used in too high a concentration it may cause sensitisation in a small proportion of people.

rosemary

Rosamarinus officinalis: *From the plant family Lamiaceae (Labiatae)*

Comes mainly from Mediterranean countries like Spain, France, Italy and Tunisia but is grown the world over.

The oil is made from the leaves and flowers of the herb.

Properties claimed for Rosemary essential oil include: Analgesic, antiseptic, antispasmodic, antiviral, astringent, cephalic, diuretic, hypotensive, rubefacient, stimulant, nervine, vulnerary, cordial, tonic and uplifting.

Summary: Rosemary comes from the same plant family as Lavender and shares many of its properties and usage.

History: Rosemary has a long and rich history which stretches back as far as the Ancient Greeks. They used it to purify the air and to prevent airborne infections and viruses. They also spread sprigs of the herb on floors to deter vermin. Dioscorides recommended its use for stomach and liver problems whilst Hippocrates suggested using Rosemary in cooking when combatting liver and spleen disorders.

Romans revered Rosemary as a sacred plant. Traces of Rosemary have also been found in Egyptian tombs. During the Middle Ages it was used to ward off devils during exorcisms and it was burned as a fumigant in sick rooms for many centuries. Indeed, the French continued to burn it in hospitals into the 21st century.

Modern research has proved the antiseptic action of Rosemary so the use of the plant to ward off the plague during the Middle Ages makes more sense now than it probably did at the time!

It continues to be one of the most popular oils used in Aromatherapy to this day. It's also found in many commercially available shampoos, soaps, shower gels, cosmetics and detergents.

Usage & methods of application: Rosemary is an essential oil which can contain different properties and constituents depending on where in the world the plant used to produce it has been grown. These are known as "chemotypes" and Rosemary comes in three types. Borneol is a particularly stimulating version and is best for relaxing muscles and in massage treatments aimed at easing problems with the liver or kidneys. Cineol is best for inhalations and is clearing and soothing for problems with the sinuses.

Heightened rejuvenating abilities can be found in the verbonene type which is considered best for skincare blends. Confusingly all three are still known as Rosmarinus Officinalis but we recommend that you ensure you are aware of which strain you are purchasing.

When burned or vaporised Rosemary acts to protect against and lessen the symptoms of flu, colds, chest infections and sinusitis. It also works on the mental side to clear the mind, refreshing and activating the brain to help bring mental clarity. It may also help those suffering from fatigue, lethargy and works to improve the memory.

In massage Rosemary is recognised as a stimulating oil and is commonly found in preparations for exercise related injuries and pains. It may also assist the treatment of arthritis, rheumatism and bursitis. It's a rubefacient and so stimulates poor circulation and can help to improve low blood pressure.

Rosemary can also be used in hair treatments. It's thought to be effective against dandruff and some even claim that it can assist in renewing hair growth and prevent premature balding. It's a great oil to use in the morning shower as it stimulates the brain and gets you going for the day.

Rosemary is a lovely to oil to burn or vaporise. You get the physical and mental benefit of the vapour from the oil as well as a gorgeous aroma.

It should be diluted in a carrier oil before use in massage. For the best results, dilute to 5% or less and massage the affected area in a circular motion.

Like many essential oils, Rosemary can be added to other cosmetic and toiletry products to make use of its wonderful properties. For example, to take advantage of its positive effect on the hair and scalp, simply add a drop or two to your existing shampoo and shake the bottle thoroughly before each use.

Blends well with: All essential oils generally blend well with one another. You may find that Rosemary blends particularly well with Cedarwood, Citronella, Geranium, Lavender, Lemongrass and Peppermint.

Toxicity & safety: Rosemary essential oil should be avoided by pregnant or breast feeding women as well as by those with epilepsy or high blood pressure.

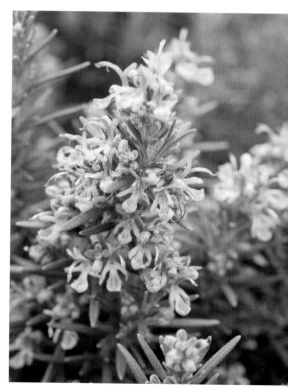

sage

Salvia officinalis: *From the plant family Lamiaceae (Labiatae).*

Native to Mediterranean countries, now cultivated the world over especially in Spain, Turkey, Greece, Italy, France and the USA amongst others.

The oil is obtained by steam distillation of the leaves of the herb.

Properties claimed for Sage essential oil include: Anti-inflammatory, antimicrobial, anti-oxidant, antiseptic, antispasmodic, astringent, digestive, diuretic, emmenagogue, febrifuge, insecticidal, stomachic and tonic.

Summary: Sage is an extremely powerful oil which should be used with great care (if at all) due to the high proportion of thujone. This can cause epileptic fits or convulsions and is toxic to the central nervous system.

History: Highly valued by the Chinese and other civilisations, Sage became revered for providing great longevity. The Chinese used to trade with the Dutch – 3 chests of tea for 1 chest of Sage. The Romans were so enamoured with the herb that specialist Sage pickers were created. They had to wear a white tunic and ensure their feet were as clean as possible before they were allowed to cultivate the plant.

Sage was one of a number of plants used in combination to ward off the plague in the Middle-Ages.

Nowadays it's occasionally found in pharmaceutical products such as mouthwash, gargles and toothpastes. Found as a fragrance in many soaps, shampoos and other personal grooming products. Extensively used as a flavouring in many food and drinks.

Usage & methods of application: Most aromatherapists use Clary Sage or another oil instead of Sage in massage and skincare as there are much safer alternatives. Please ensure you read the safety information below before using Sage essential oil.

Sage is sometimes used in massage for people with well-developed muscles as it's a muscle softener and so is used to help avoid sprains and strains.

It is very occasionally burned or vaporised to improve the memory and speed of thought and to help with depression or grief.

Blends well with: Most essential oils blend well with one another. You may find that Sage essential oil blends especially well with Bergamot, Lavender, Lemon and Rosemary.

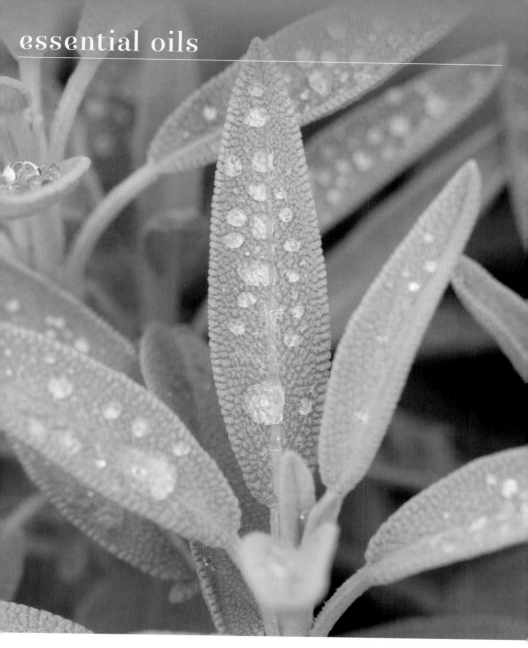

Toxicity & safety: Sage should be completely avoided by pregnant and nursing mothers, epileptics or those with high blood pressure. Extreme caution should be employed when using Sage. If you are going to use it in any blend to go on the skin it should be extremely well diluted to a maximum of 1%.

Sandalwood Amyris

Amyris balsamifera: *From the plant family Rutaceae.*

Originally from the West Indies, now found in many tropical countries all over the world including Haiti, Jamaica and South and Central America.

The oil is obtained by steam distillation of the bark of the tree.

Properties claimed for Sandalwood Amyris include: Antiseptic, balsamic and sedative.

Summary: Whilst not a true Sandalwood, Amyris shares some of the same properties and is often used as a cheaper and more ethically sound substitute.

History: Not much is known of the history of Amyris but it was used by Haitians (particularly fishermen and traders) as a torch due to the high percentage of oil in the wood. They called it Candle Wood. The wood is also popular in furniture making.

Usage & methods of application: The main use of Amyris in Aromatherapy is as a fixative in blends to help accentuate the aroma of other oils. It's also used in massage blends aimed at relaxing and soothing muscles whilst in skincare blends it's used to moisturise and soften dry and irritated skin.

When burned or vaporised Amyris is good oil to use in a blend to add a woody note to the aroma. It's a calming oil and is sometimes found in blends for meditation.

Blends well with: Most essential oils blend well with one another. You may find that Amyris blends particularly well with Clary Sage, Geranium, Ylang Ylang, Galbanum, Lavender, Benzoin and Frankincense.

Toxicity & safety: Generally regarded as non-toxic and non-irritant, Amyris should be avoided by pregnant and nursing mothers just to be on the safe side.

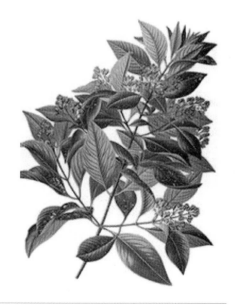

essential oils

tea tree

Melalueca alternifolia: From the plant family Myrtaceae.
Originates from Australia.
The oil is made from the twigs and leaves of the Tea Tree.
Extracted by steam distillation.
Properties claimed for Tea Tree essential oil include: Anti-inflammatory, antiseptic, antiviral, bactericidal, cooling, fungicidal, immuno-stimulant, sudorific, vulnerary, tonic.

Summary: Tea Tree is one of the few oils proven to have an effect on the three main types of infection to which humans are susceptible – bacteria, viruses and fungi. This makes it the number 1 oil to have in your first aid box – it's useful for the prevention and the treatment of infections and is suitable for application to minor cuts and abrasions.

Australian Aborigines have utilised the amazing disinfectant and antibacterial properties of Tea Tree oil for thousands of years to treat all manner of ailments from throat infections to coughs, colds and as a general antiseptic. Modern medical research has confirmed Tea Tree to be hugely effective when correctly used.

History: Tea Tree has an interesting history having swung in and out of fashion over the years.

As mentioned above, the Aborigines of the New South Wales coast had been using the oil for thousands of years with extremely positive results. The first Europeans to encounter Tea Tree were James Cook and the crew of the HMS Endeavour when they landed on the Australian coast in 1770.

Cook is actually the man responsible for naming the plant 'Tea Tree'. He witnessed the natives brewing the leaves in much the same way as his servants on the boat would have made tea for drinking and thus the name was established.

Then in 1923 a man called Arthur Penfold decided to properly test the oil in an attempt to understand why it worked so well. He showed that it was 12 times more potent than Carbolic Acid, the most commonly used antiseptic of the day.

His work lead to further clinical studies in Europe and throughout the following decades Tea Tree was written about very positively in the most respected medical journals. Australian soldiers were issued with

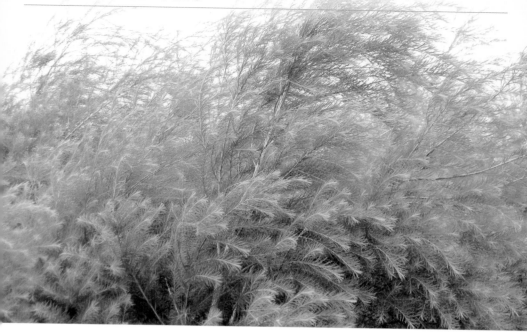

a bottle of Tea Tree in their first aid kits and the oil also began to appear in shampoos and toothpastes as well as treatments for lice, smelly feet, boils and acne.

Like a lot of natural remedies, Tea Tree was sidelined by developments in cheaper, mass produced synthetic medicine which soon became the default option for medical practitioners. The Tea Tree industry suffered and pretty much collapsed altogether in the 1960s.

Times were tough for Tea Tree producers until the late 1970s when people once again realised the power of nature could be harnessed to produce a mass market product. John White was in the vanguard of the new movement. A cameraman by trade, he realised that there would be a demand for a natural, effective oil like Tea Tree and set up a plantation.

It took 4 years to produce the first oil. Sadly, White's health failed and he was unable to complete the project that he had started. His stepson Michael White took over the business and he and other producers saw Tea Tree return once again to popular use.

Today Tea Tree is used worldwide for its natural properties and its popularity is still increasing as more and more people become aware of the benefits of this fantastic natural product.

Usage & methods of application:
(For safe usage please refer to the Safety and Toxicity section below). Tea Tree has a huge abundance of potential uses thanks to its many health giving properties. In general terms Tea Tree is used to boost the immune system and so minimise the amount time

a person is ill because it is thought to enhance the body's natural defences. It can also be useful in readying the body ahead of an operation as well as improving recovery post-op.

It's used to treat dermatological conditions such as athlete's foot, psoriasis and eczema. It's effective against lice and because it attacks the Propionibacterium acnes and Staphylococcus aureus bacteria which cause acne and boils respectively, it's commonly found in blends for these skin problems too.

Scientific studies have proven the effectiveness of Tea Tree oil in these treatments and have also shown that Tea Tree disperses infectious material and debris trapped within a wound.

It's also a wonderful multi-purpose oil to keep handy at home. Because of its antibacterial action, Tea Tree works extremely well when applied to minor cuts and abrasions, stings, mosquito and other insect bites as well as rashes and burns including sunburn. The anti-fungal, anti-viral and strong antiseptic properties of the oil make it one of the best natural remedies available.

Tea Tree is good in massage as a treatment for sore and achy muscles and is also found in soaps, toothpastes (it attacks the bacteria that cause gingivitis and cavities), skin washing preparations and deodorants.

It's especially effective against fungal infections such as athlete's foot and vaginal infections and is the perfect treatment for infected toe nails. It can

be helpful in the treatment of warts, verrucae and cold sores.

It can also be beneficial in hair care. Tea Tree has been shown to regulate sebum production meaning it can not only help to soothe and cure dry, flaky skin (and the dandruff that results from these issues) but can also correct overly oily hair.

It's also suggested that Tea Tree may be instrumental in the attempts to control virulent infections such as MRSA. Bugs like this one have become resistant to synthetic antibiotics as these man made substances are developed to only attack microorganisms in a specific way. Once the microorganisms have learned to thwart these attacks they pass on the information to their offspring and it becomes a never ending battle between the mutating cells and the scientists.

Tea Tree may be an answer as because it's a natural product it attacks the whole organism and so is less likely to be defeated by bacteria. There is also research being undertaken to determine the effectiveness of Tea Tree in treating skin cancers.

Before you use Tea Tree or any essential oil please ensure that you are familiar with the contraindications. You should also perform a skin patch test before application to the rest of your body to ensure no sensitisation occurs.

Tea Tree can be used neat on the skin but only in very small amounts and great care should be taken before application. If you are unsure please consult a professional aromatherapist or a doctor. Tea Tree oil should never be swallowed or taken internally.

essential oils

A dab of Tea Tree on acne or a boil twice a day can help to clear up any problems – Tea Tree is a strong, natural antiseptic. Simply add a drop or two to a clean tissue and apply to the affected area.

Its antiviral and anti-bacterial properties make it a preferred natural treatment for athlete's foot – again, one drop applied to the affected area in the morning and the evening should soon help to clear up most cases.

Try adding a drop to your shampoo to combat dandruff or head lice. Place the amount of shampoo you normally use in the palm of your hand, add a drop of Tea Tree and lather well before application. It can also help with greasy, oily and dry scalps and hair as it balances the production of sebum.

Tea Tree works very well in a vaporiser to protect from airborne viruses and bacteria. It's also worth burning or inhaling once the lurgy has set in as it helps to improve recovery times. It is also effective against sinus problems when used in this way.

This versatile oil can also be very useful around the house. You can create your own, simple natural cleaning fluid by mixing 2-3 drops of Tea Tree in 100 or 200ml of water in a bottle with a spray attachment. Make sure you shake the bottle well before each use and then spray on to surfaces and tables in the same way as you would with any other spray cleaner. This solution not only cleans but also protects thanks to the bactericidal and antiviral properties of the oil.

Used this way Tea Tree can banish mould, keep germs away from kids car seats and high chairs and, when added to salt, makes a great way to scrub clean tiles, bathtubs and sinks.

We think every household should have a bottle of Tea Tree somewhere. It has so many uses both in treatment and around the home that a house is empty without a bottle of Tea Tree!

Blends well with: All essential oils generally blend well with one another. You may find that Tea Tree blends particularly well with Cinnamon, Clary Sage, Clove, Geranium, Lavender, Lemon, Myrrh, Nutmeg, Rosewood, Rosemary and Thyme.

Toxicity & safety: Tea Tree should never be taken internally. Areas around the eyes, ears and nose should also be avoided. It's a generally safe oil for external application but care should always be taken as it can irritate the skin in some cases.

There are no specific indications to suggest that pregnant or nursing mothers should avoid Tea Tree but if you are concerned then it would be advisable to speak with your midwife or a qualified aromatherapist.

ylang ylang

Cananga odorata: *From the plant family Annonaceae.*

Native to Asia, especially the Philippines and Indonesia. Now produced in many countries but mainly Madagascar, Comoro Islands & Reunion.

Obtained by steam distillation of the flowers.

Properties claimed for Ylang Ylang essential oil include: Aphrodisiac, antidepressant, antiseptic, euphoric, hypotensive, sedative, stimulant and tonic.

Summary: People either love or hate Ylang Ylang but it always provokes strong feelings one way or the other. Regarded as a natural aphrodisiac and as a soothing oil.

History: Ylang Ylang oil is obtained from the tree of the same name. It takes 5 years for each tree to mature before the oil can be distilled. However, once established a healthy tree can produce up to 45 pounds of raw material per annum for as long as 50 years. It takes around 50 pounds of raw material to produce roughly 1 litre of essential oil.

Ylang Ylang has long been considered one of the most romantic of plants and oils. This is due to the well-recognised aphrodisiac properties of the oil. In Indonesia, the petals of the flowers are spread on the bed of newly married couples on their wedding night. It's also long been popular in massage blends for people looking to ignite a romantic spark.

The Filipinos use the oil to treat cuts, burns, grazes and bites from both insects and snakes. Asian cultures have used Ylang Ylang for thousands of years to calm a distressed heart.

In the 20th century two French scientists carried out a series of experiments using Ylang Ylang and confirmed that it's a great oil for steadying the heart. They also found that it was very useful in the treatments of several serious diseases including malaria and typhus.

Nowadays Ylang Ylang can be found in many soaps, cosmetics and perfumes. It's mainly used for its perfume and as a fixative. It's also found in food and drinks both soft and alcoholic as a flavouring. It provides the top note in one of the world's most popular perfumes (Chanel No.5) as well as many other well-known scents.

Usage & methods of application: Ylang Ylang should always be used in small amounts as it has a strong aroma and potent properties which can easily overpower other oils in your blend.

When blended for massage Ylang Ylang is often found in preparations used to

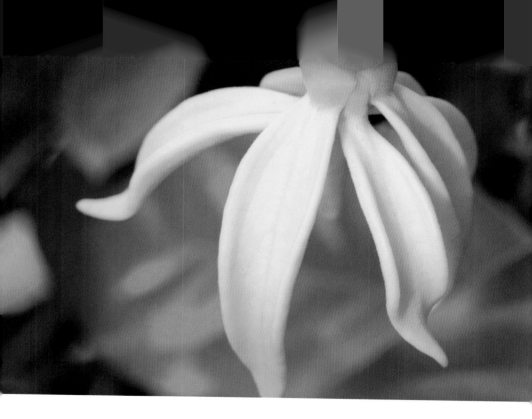

treat high blood pressure, tachycardia, unusually fast breathing and palpitations. It's both calming and uplifting so is often found in blends to relieve depression, insomnia, nervous tension and stress related problems.

It's also commonly used as an ingredient in sensual blends designed for home use. A romantic oil which is a natural aphrodisiac and is also thought to discourage frigidity and assist in the relief of impotence.

In a cream or lotion it is used to alleviate oily, irritated skin, insect bites and stings, acne and is regarded as a good general skin tonic.

When burned or vaporised it is again used to set a romantic mood and also to alleviate depression and fatigue. It can also be helpful in encouraging the body to expel mucous and to calm exaggerated coughing fits.

Blends well with: Most essential oils blend well with one another. You may find that Ylang Ylang blends especially well with Bergamot, Grapefruit, Lavender and Sandalwood.

Toxicity & safety: Generally non-toxic and non-irritant although it may cause sensitisation to the skin in a few individuals. It should be used in small amounts as it has a strong aroma which can invoke headaches or nausea in some people. In very rare cases Ylang Ylang can induce epileptic seizures.

absolute & precious oils

calendula

Calendula officinalis: From the plant family Asteraceae.
Thought to be native to Southern Europe.
Obtained by ethanolic and solvent extraction of the whole plant.
Properties claimed for Calendula include: Tonic, emmenagogue,
antispasmodic, anti-oxidant, anti-inflammatory, anti-microbial and sudorific.

Summary: Regarded as a soothing and calming oil, Calendula is probably
best known for its anti-inflammatory action and is commonly found in
preparations for the skin.

History: Calendula has been used for medicinal, spiritual and culinary purposes for thousands of years. It was traditionally used as a salve combined with goat's cheese for sunburn, bruises and other burns (it's still used for these purposes today but is not normally combined with the goat's cheese!). It was used during the American Civil War to treat wounds, whilst elsewhere poultices of Calendula were used to treat smallpox.

In the 16th and 17th centuries many herbalists wrote about the perceived medical benefits of Calendula. It was used to treat headaches, jaundice, red-eye, problems with the skin and toothache among other ailments.

Usage & methods of application:
When blended with a base oil, cream or lotion Calendula is often found in preparations for dry, dehydrated, irritated and rough skin as well as in cases of broken capillaries. It's often used as an ingredient in general healing blends as well as blends targeted at healing wounds, eczema and to fight signs of ageing.

Calendula in cream is often used to relieve sore and cracked nipples in breastfeeding women and when blended in a lotion it can be used as a soothing and protecting massage for babies and infants.

Additionally it's used in treatments for acne and the anti-microbial and anti-oxidising properties make it popular in blends to fight infection while a drop of the oil in a bath is sometimes recommended for psoriasis.

Blends well with: Most essential oils blend well with one another. You may find that Calendula blends especially well with Lavender, Frankincense, Cypress and Bergamot.

Safety & toxicity: Generally considered to be a safe oil for use on the skin.

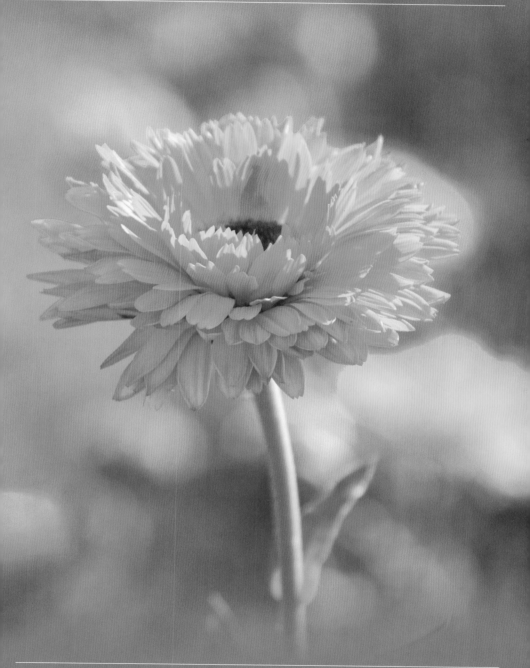

jasmin

Jasminum officinale: *From the plant family Oleaceae.*

Commonly found the world over. There is confusion over where the plant was originally found but most people agree that it's native to central Asia.

The oil is obtained by solvent extraction from the flowers.

Properties claimed for Jasmin include: Antidepressant, antispasmodic, aphrodisiac, relaxing, sedative and tonic.

Summary: A rejuvenating oil for both the skin and the soul. Relaxing, soothing and uplifting – also known as the "King of Oils".

History: An ancient plant with a history that reaches back thousands of years. The name comes from the Persian word Yasmin (fragrant flower). It's believed that it was introduced to Ancient Egypt in around 1000 BC and for hundreds of years it was the preserve of the rich and privileged in Egypt, India and the Orient. Indeed, it was worshipped by Chinese emperors. It's thought that this was due to its perceived aphrodisiac properties.

It was introduced to Europe in the 17th century after being brought to Spain by the Moors. It quickly spread from Spain to the rest of Europe and was a highly fashionable item for the next couple of hundred years.

Jasmin has come to symbolise different things in many cultures but they all have one thing in common – the theme of love, desire or hope. It symbolises "divine hope" in India, represents the sweetness of women in China and is regarded as the perfume of love in Hindu and Muslim cultures.

The Chinese also used various parts of the plant to treat hepatitis, cirrhosis of the liver, headaches, insomnia, rheumatism and dysentery.

Jasmin flowers are best picked in the evening as the fragrance of the flowers actually reduces in sunlight. It takes around 1000lbs of Jasmin flowers to produce roughly 1 litre of oil.

In modern times Jasmin remains a highly popular oil in perfumery and other cosmetics, soaps and toiletries. The oil is also used in many food and drink products and the dried flowers are used to make the popular Jasmin tea.

Usage & methods of application:
When blended in a carrier oil or lotion Jasmin is often used in skincare for dry, greasy, sensitive or irritated skin. It can also be used to alleviate sore muscles, spasms and sprains and is considered to be soothing for menstrual pain and attendant emotional issues. It's also used in sensual massage blends to create an atmosphere of love and lust.

absolute & precious oils

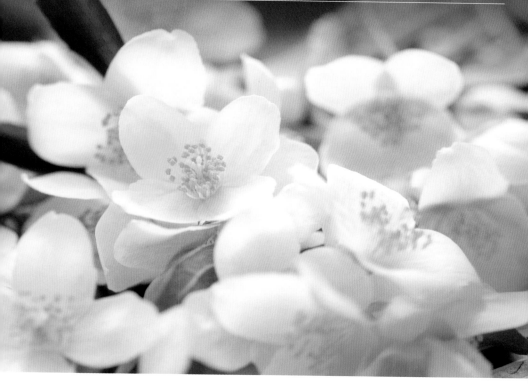

For a more intense romantic atmosphere you could combine a massage with the burning or vaporising of Jasmin too. It's also used in this way to relieve frigidity, depression, nervous exhaustion and many stress-related issues and also to promote confidence, optimism and even euphoria.

Jasmin is also becoming more and more popular as one of the essential oils used during natural childbirth. As increasing numbers of people choose to forego the use of synthetic chemical drugs as they bring new life into the world and instead use natural pain relief, Jasmin is thought to strengthen contractions, relieve pain in the uterus and also assist with recovery after the birth.

Blends well with: Most essential oils blend well with one another. You may find that Jasmin blends especially well with Rose oils, Sandalwood, Clary Sage and all the citrus oils.

Safety & toxicity: Non-toxic, non-irritant and generally non-sensitising although it can cause sensitisation in some individuals so caution is advised. It should not be used by pregnant women. It's advisable to use Jasmin in small quantities as over-exposure can affect concentration due to the powerful relaxing properties of the oil.

neroli

Citrus Aurantium: *From the plant family Rutaceae.*

Native to China and Central Asia, now grown, cultivated and distilled in North Africa, China and most Mediterranean countries.

The oil is obtained by distillation and solvent extraction.

Properties claimed for Neroli include: Antidepressant, antispasmodic, detoxifying, relaxing, sedative, tonic and uplifting.

Summary: A wonderfully rejuvenating and uplifting oil which uplifts both the body and the mind.

History: Neroli first came to prominence in the Far East and was later introduced to the West by Arabian traders.

It made it to the Mediterranean region of Spain by the 12th century and plantations soon appeared here and in other nearby countries with a suitable climate. These plantations were cultivated to produce the essential oil. The oil was soon in high demand and became extremely popular with the great and the not so good of the time including several royal families around Europe.

It was worn to scent articles of clothing such as gloves, not only giving a beautiful aroma but also acting to calm the nerves. For this reason the blossom was often included in the bouquets carried by brides in Europe. It was also used to decorate the hair of brides and was placed next to the marital bed to proclaim their virginity and calm any wedding nerves. This tradition still continues today in parts of southern Europe.

Neroli is still present in around 12% of modern high quality perfumes, a trend started in the 1700s by the Italian perfumer J.M. Farina who created a blend using Neroli, Lavender, Bergamot, Petitgrain, Lemon and Rosemary which he called Eau de Cologne.

In modern times Neroli is used to flavour many pharmaceuticals, foods and drinks. The absolute is commonly found in the higher end perfumes, Eau de Colognes and toilet waters.

Usage & methods of application: When blended for massage, Neroli is often used in skincare to treat stretch marks, scars, mature and sensitive skin, wrinkles, varicose veins and to tone the complexion. It's often regarded as the mature woman's best friend. It's also found in blends aimed at easing palpitations and to improve circulation as well as in the treatment of stomach issues such as excessive flatulence, spasms and dyspepsia caused by nerves.

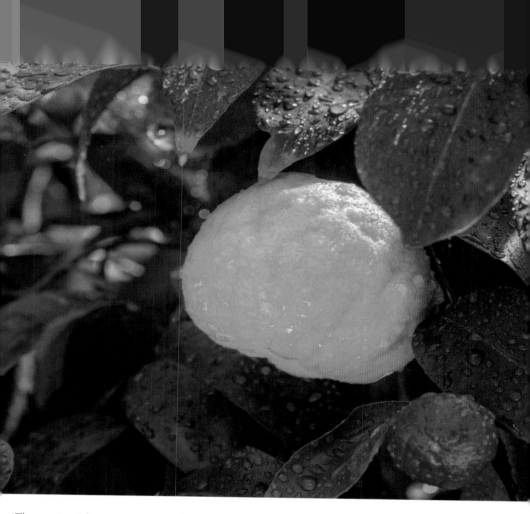

The anti-oxidant properties of the oil can encourage cell growth which in turn can boost dull and oily hair and return it to a healthier condition. It can also be helpful in relieving an irritated scalp as well as dermatitis in general. You just need to add some to a shampoo or conditioner base – around 5-7 drops of the absolute per 100ml of the base ingredient.

It's most often burned or vaporised for its beautiful aroma and also to calm, relax and de-stress as well as in cases of insomnia, anxiety and depression.

Blends well with: Essential oils generally blend well with one another. You may find that Neroli blends especially well with Chamomile, Geranium, Coriander, Clary Sage, Jasmine, Lavender, Rose, Ylang Ylang, Coriander and the Citrus oils.

Safety & toxicity: A very safe oil, Neroli is non-toxic, non-irritant, non-sensitising and non-phototoxic.

rose maroc

Rosa centifolia: *From the plant family Rosaceae.*

The absolute is obtained by alcohol extraction from the concrete.

Properties claimed for Rose Maroc include: Antidepressant, antiseptic, antispasmodic, antiviral, aphrodisiac, bactericidal, emmenagogue, laxative, sedative and tonic.

Summary: One of the most relaxing of all the Rose oils with great skincare properties too. Also a noted aphrodisiac.

History: Roses are believed to have first been cultivated in Persia but are now mainly produced in Morocco, Tunisia, France and China.

Roses have been used in many cultures since ancient times. Highly prized by the Greeks, Chinese, Indians, Persians and Romans and used for numerous treatments such as nervous tension, headaches, liver complaints, fever, digestive problems, issues with menstruation, poor circulation and skin complaints. Rose Maroc has also been used in sensual preparations due to its reputation as an aphrodisiac.

Rose is one of the most favoured oils used in perfumery and is still found in a high percentage of fragrances for both men and women today. It's also commonly found in soaps, cosmetics, toiletries and as a flavouring agent in food, drink and tobacco products.

Usage & methods of application:
In Aromatherapy skincare Rose is often blended with other oils in a carrier oil and used in cases of broken capillaries, dry skin, eczema, wrinkles and is especially beneficial to mature and sensitive skin. It's also used in Aromatherapy massage to improve circulation, calm palpitations and to ease tension and stress related conditions. It may also be used in cases of asthma and hay fever and to improve the digestive system, ease nausea and congestion of the liver.

When burned or vaporised it's used as an uplifting oil and is often recommended in cases of depression, frigidity, impotence, insomnia, nervous tension and stress.

Blends well with: Most essential oils blend well with one another. You may find that Rose Maroc blends especially well with Neroli, Lavender, Bergamot, Clary Sage, Sandalwood, Patchouli, Benzoin, Palmarosa, Clove and Chamomile.

Safety & toxicity: Non-sensitising, non-toxic and non-irritant with no known contraindications. It's probably best avoided during pregnancy.

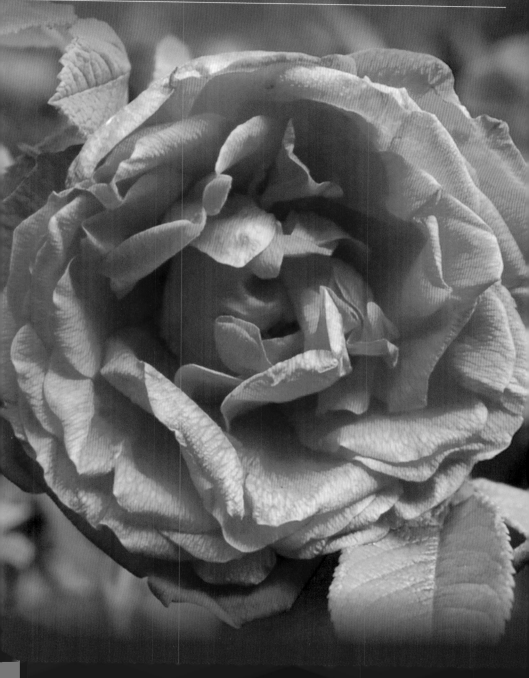

rose otto steam distilled

Rosa damascena: *From the plant family Rosaceae.*

Thought to originate from the Orient, now mainly cultivated in Bulgaria, France and Turkey.

Obtained by steam distillation of the petals of the flower.

Properties claimed for Rose Otto include: Antidepressant, antiseptic, antispasmodic, antiviral, aphrodisiac, astringent, bactericidal, emmenagogue, haemostatic, hepatic, laxative, nervous system sedative, stomachic and tonic for the heart, liver, stomach and uterus.

Summary: Also known as Damask Rose, it's regarded as particularly effective in aiding problems of an emotional and reproductive nature as well as being a noted aphrodisiac. It's one of the more expensive oils, however only a small amount is needed to make a big difference to a blend so it's worth the investment.

History: Rose Otto has a somewhat confused history with differing claims as to the eventual distribution of the oil. It's actually a hybrid and is thought to have originated in the Middle East (some claim specifically the Gulf of Persia). There are three main theories as to how it spread to the rest of the world. One theory claims that the Crusader Robert De Brie brought it from Syria to Europe in the middle part of the 13th century, others claim the Romans were responsible for bringing it from the Middle East and a third theory is that a physician gave it to Henry VIII as a gift in around 1540.

It is generally agreed that Persia (now Iran) was the epicentre of the cultivation of the plant for 700 years between the 10th and 17th centuries. The industry gradually spread outwards from Persia to Arabia, Palestine, Greece, India, North Africa and was taken as far as Spain by the Moors.

Turkish Ottoman merchants imported the plant to the Balkan countries sometime during the 16th century and it was at this time that it was introduced to Bulgaria. A new town was founded in Bulgaria called Kazanlik which translates as "the place of stills" and it was here that new cultivations were centred. It was near a valley which provided the perfect growing conditions and eventually the oil produced here became regarded as the finest available. The area became known as "The Valley of the Roses" and Bulgarian growers dominated the market from the 19th century until around the time of WW2.

Turkey then got heavily involved in the cultivation and farming of the plant and

absolute & precious oils

it's thought that the Turks now produce more Rose Otto than anyone else. Opinions vary as to where the finest oil is produced but it's generally considered that Bulgaria still just about holds the edge in terms of quality if not quantity.

The roses are still harvested by hand and are collected at sunrise as soon as the flowers start to open. The harvesting continues each day until the dew disappears from the plant and is continued over a few weeks until every single flower has been picked.

Rose petals were traditionally used to ensure a long and happy marriage – the petals being spread on the floor during weddings. Rose Otto is still used today in meditation and prayer and remains a symbol of love and purity in many cultures. It was also used for menstrual, digestive and circulation problems as well as in incense and perfumes.

Today it's found in many perfumes, toiletries, soaps and cosmetics as well as being occasionally used as a flavouring in food products.

It takes 60 roses to produce 1 drop of Rose Otto oil which will help you to understand why this oil is so expensive!

Usage & methods of application:
An uplifting oil, Rose Otto is often blended with a carrier oil and/or other essential oils for massage to help alleviate stress, nervous tension, depression, grief, baby blues, problems associated with allergies and headaches or migraine. It may also be used as a skin treatment, especially for mature, dry or sensitive skin – it's often added to a base cream or lotion for these purposes too. Additionally it's used to treat broken capillaries, redness of the skin and inflammations. It's an astringent oil which makes it a great general tonic for the skin.

When burned or vaporised it's again mainly used as an uplifting oil and is particularly recommended in times of grief, to calm anger and lift depression. It can help to calm an overly busy mind and may also be used to alleviate respiratory problems too.

Blends well with: Most essential oils blend well with one another. However, you may find that Rose Otto blends especially well with Geranium, Palmarosa, Clove, Jasmin, Patchouli, Mimosa, Lavender, Benzoin and Chamomile.

Toxicity & safety: Non-toxic, non-sensitising and non-irritant, Rose Otto is generally regarded as a safe oil but should be avoided during pregnancy nonetheless.

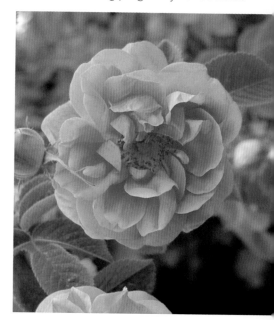

carrier oils

carrier oils

Being so concentrated, essential oils are always diluted into a base preparation before applying to the skin. These can range from nut or vegetable oils through to everyday toiletries, such as shampoos and conditioners.

argan

(Argania spinosa)

Indigenous to Morocco, Argan Oil is cold pressed from the kernels of the Argan tree fruit which look a little like oversized olives. In its virgin state it has a nutty aroma though some manufacturers remove the odour to make it more adaptable within blends and preparations.

Its historic uses in Morocco span from culinary to skin and haircare. The popularity of Argan Oil has become more widespread due to its inclusion in hair products; however these benefits can be easily reaped by adding it to homemade blends.

It is deeply moisturising, readily absorbed and excellent for face, body and hair treatments. It contains Vitamin A, B1, B2, B6 and E and can help protect and regenerate even the most sensitive of skins.

Argan Oil's soothing and healing properties work particularly well on the delicate skin around the eyes, neck and décolletage, over time reversing signs of ageing. For hair, it is perfect for masks and makes a good, light finishing oil when applied to the tips.

avocado

(Persea gratissima)

Deep green in colour with a naturally occurring odour, avocado oil is made by pressing the dried flesh of the avocado fruit. The flesh and oil possess a rich profile of Vitamins E, B5 and lecithin, beta-carotene, plant sterols and chlorophyll.

As an indigenous plant of Central and South America it has been used for centuries for skin and haircare as well as being an important, nourishing part of the traditional diet. The cold pressed oil is thick and viscous yet is absorbed deeply by skin.

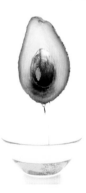

If it feels too 'tacky' just lighten the texture by adding a shorter base oil such as grapeseed or evening primrose. The benefit of its heavier viscosity is that it can be used to thicken lotions and creams. Skin types best matched to Avocado are dry, mature and in need of deep nourishment and they tend to drink up this type of nutrient rich carrier oil.

carrier oils

argan

evening primrose

(Oenethera biennis)

The oil is cold pressed from the tiny seeds of the delicate yellow flower of the Evening Primrose which is native to North America. As with many plant species its healing properties have been utilised for years by indigenous peoples and then naturalised around the world where the climate and habitat suited its growth.

Known most commonly as a dietary supplement, Evening Primrose has many benefits when applied topically. It has a high count of gamma linoleic acid (GLA) which helps the body combat conditions related to inflammation, premenstrual tension and high blood pressure.

With a very light and easily absorbed consistency Evening Primrose Oil can be used alone and also can be added to other carriers which would increase the blend's moisturising effect.

Due to its GLA content it can be used to shrink open pores on combination to greasy skin types and can help soothe inflamed acne-prone skin. It can seem counter intuitive to apply oils to oily skin but the benefits will be plain to see and feel within a couple of weeks.

Evening Primrose can also help soothe eczema, soften dry and scaly skin, speed up wound healing, and help alleviate dandruff.

grapeseed

(Vitis vinifera)

Extracted from the seeds of grapes, most grapeseed oil is produced in countries with a well-established wine making industry. It is of a light consistency, absorbing into the skin rapidly but leaving very little residue, making it a good option for quick application.

Grapeseed Oil is often the first choice as a nut-free carrier and is always used for baby massage. Its chemical make-up includes a high percentage of linoleic acid, known as omega 6, a crucial element in aiding the body to regulate inflammation.

Grapeseed Oil is a good choice of carrier oil when treating circulatory problems because it strengthens vein health and skin that has traces of atrophy (thinning) due to hydrocortisone cream usage. It is also excellent for combination to greasy skin types with its slightly astringent properties and ability to reduce pore size if used for a prolonged period.

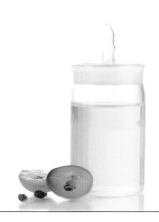

jojoba

(Buxus chinensis)

Unique amongst the carriers, Jojoba is a liquid wax rather than an oil. Native to the South Western deserts of North America it has been used by tribes of the region for wound, skin and haircare.

Jojoba has a very similar structure to the skin's natural oil, known as sebum. If skin is too dry it can be due to a lack of sebum. Conversely, over-production of sebum can lead to a greasy complexion.

Jojoba can help both ends of the skin spectrum and is particularly useful to acne-prone skins due to its myristic acid content. This is naturally occurring within Jojoba and has wonderful anti-inflammatory, anti-fungal and antibacterial properties. Again, it may seem odd to apply a liquid wax to greasy skin but within a fortnight the results will be clear.

Alongside these qualities, Jojoba is a popular choice for any situation where staying power is required. It works well for face and hair masks, as a base for scented perfume oils and can thicken any lotion or cream base.

rosehip

(Rosa Canina)

Extracted from the tiny seeds within the ripened rosehips this light, easily absorbed oil is often used as the base for facial oils. Its regenerative effect on skin has been much researched within Chile, where the oil has been extremely popular for many years.

Studies show that it is useful in reducing and even reversing fine lines, UV exposure and scars. Its light texture is perfect for use on the face and can be used on any skin type where a little extra help is needed.

Rosehip has a high Vitamin A count which protects and repairs the skin whilst naturally occurring Vitamin C boosts the skin's ability to produce collagen, maintaining a firmness and freshness.

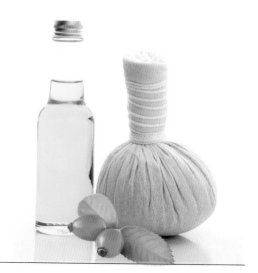

sweet almond

(Prunus amygdalus dulcis)

Sweet Almond Oil has been used since antiquity around the Mediterranean basin where the trees were first cultivated in around 3000BC. To this day it is a very popular choice and the most commonly used carrier oil for general skincare and massage.

Cold pressed from the kernels, it contains a combination of vitamins A, B1, B2 and E as well as monounsaturated, polyunsaturated and saturated fatty acids. Best suited to normal to dry skin types, it remains on the skin's surface for a moderate amount of time (depending on how much is applied), gradually absorbing to leave the skin soft and supple.

Sweet Almond can make an excellent emollient to soothe sensitive, irritated or chapped skin and is known to be non-reactive and mild on all skin types including infants. As it is a nut oil, please be aware of any potential nut allergies before using on yourself or others.

wheatgerm

(Triticum vulgare)

Popular as an addition to other base preparations, Wheatgerm Oil is extracted by warm pressing the germ of the wheat. It has a rich wheaty odour which can be a little overpowering if used alone. Wheatgerm is a viscous, sticky oil with a slow rate of absorption making it perfect in fortifying other lighter oils.

It has a very high Vitamin E content and rich in essential fatty acids which nourish dry, thirsty skin and have a healing effect on scars. Adding Wheatgerm Oil to any blend of carrier will boost its nourishing properties and is best used in the treatment of dry skin conditions as it may overload combination skin types.

carrier oils

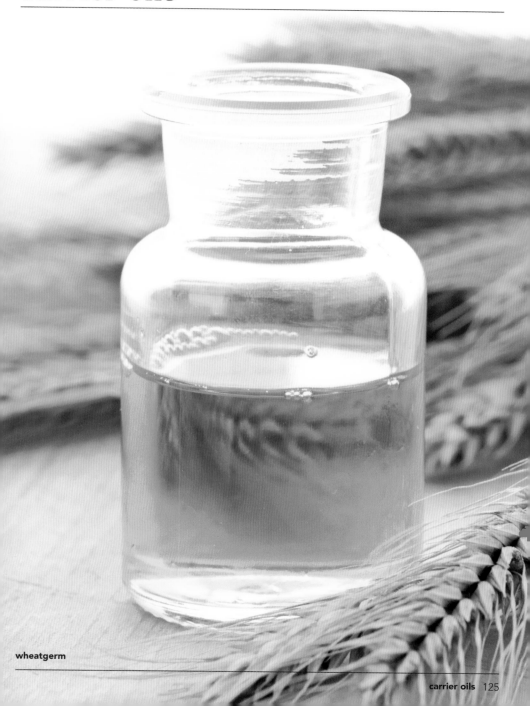

wheatgerm

floral waters

floral waters

Hydrosols and Hydrolates:
Many people use the above terms interchangeably but a clear distinction can be made between the two. Hydrosols are the result of the dissolving of essential oils in distilled water, while Hydrolates are a natural by-product of the steam distillation of essential oils. Both are extremely useful in skincare and have many other potential applications. The properties of a floral water correspond to the essential oil but at a much gentler level.

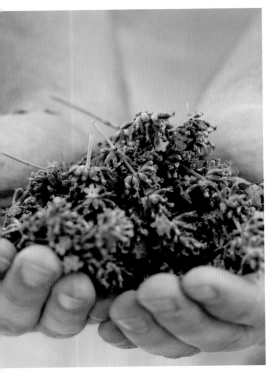

Suggested Uses: Floral Waters are most commonly used as a toner. As part of your cleansing regime, floral water applied to cotton wool can be swept over the face and neck to remove the final traces of cleanser and close the pores.

A refreshing face or body mist can be created by filling an atomiser or spray bottle with your chosen floral water. These are particularly revitalising for hot days, during flights, at work and after exercising. Whenever you feel hot and bothered a spritz of floral water can help centre and revive.

Try blending floral waters with dry clays (such as kaolin) to create a mask. This can be used on face, hair or body. It is also possible to add a drop of essential oil to boost its purifying benefits. For a face mask, simply mix a couple of teaspoons of clay powder with a splash of floral water to a smoothable consistency, apply to the face (avoiding delicate eye area), leave for 10 to 15 minutes and rinse off with warm water.

To awaken tired eyes, douse a cotton wool pad with a floral water and apply over closed eyes for around 15 minutes. The floral water will gently refresh the eyelids and surrounding area. This is the best way to treat the eyes as essential oils are too powerful for this sensitive and delicate skin.

floral waters

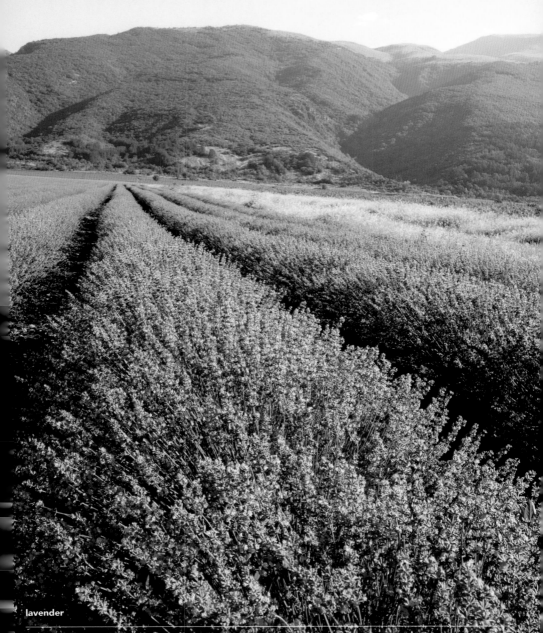

lavender

popular floral waters

chamomile

Noted for its calming, anti-inflammatory properties, chamomile is suited to easily inflamed skin conditions. This can cover eczema and psoriasis-prone skin although acne can often be related to inflammation too. Chamomile floral water is useful for eye infections and allergy related puffiness of the eye.

geranium

A sweet floral scent that belies Geranium's powerful hormone balancing properties. It is particularly useful for skin that is prone to breakouts due to hormone flucuations. Another good option for mixing with clays to draw out impurities. Excellent for improving skin tone as Geranium can have a positive effect on circulation.

jasmin

Known as the King of Flowers, Jasmin has a powerful floral scent that sits well with its ability to fortify the emotions. Its scent can seem heavy so this makes it a good choice for a scented body spray. Within skin preparations it can help soothe easily irritated skin and can be used beautifully as a toner, spritz or as a clay mask ingredient.

lavender

Almost an adaptogen for the skin, Lavender can soothe dryness yet also ease over-production of greasiness. Coupled with its mild antiseptic and cellular regenerative properties it is great for the full range of skin types. Its scent is more verdant than the oil of Lavender and can give a feeling of freshness.

neroli

With historic links to feelings of serenity, Neroli has a verdant aroma that can bring about a moment of true calm when spritzed onto the face. Its skin enhancing properties include cellular regeneration (similar to Lavender) and it works well for most skin types. A good choice of toner for combination skin types.

rose

A wonderful all-rounder with a universally adored scent. Rose has a strengthening effect on the underlying small capillaries within the skin which can help improve the tone and texture. Good quality Rose water has a soft floral scent which can have a profoundly comforting effect on the mind, promoting an instant sense of well-being.

floral waters

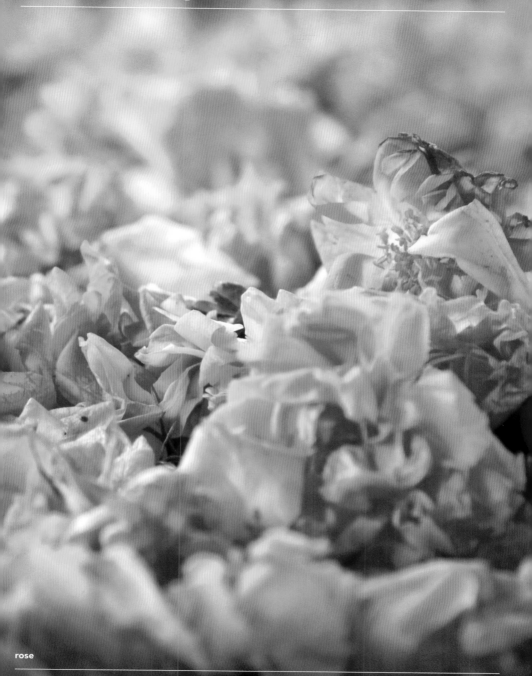

rose

physical aromatherapy

physical aromatherapy

The following recipes are made at a 5% dilution rate (5 drops of essential oils in to 5 ml of base) and are good for localised areas. If you need to create a larger batch simply multiply the ingredients accordingly. Also bear in mind your 'patient's' age, skin type and potential sensitivities and refer to the dilution rate table.

It is always good practice to conduct a sniff test of the essential oils as this will help to determine their efficiency and suitability for each individual. Don't worry if a certain oil does not resonate with the 'patient' as there is always a next best option to select from. Simply switch to a similar oil (for example, another herb or tree oil) checking that its properties will address the ailment.

Where recipes have letters in brackets next to them you should refer to the relevant method in the 'How to use essential oils' chapter.

Headaches

On set of headaches: (S) (C)
3 drops Lavender
2 drops Peppermint
5 ml Base oil or cream

Persistent headaches: (S) (C)
1 drop Lavender
1 drop Peppermint
3 drops Marjoram
5 ml Base oil or cream

Stress related headaches: (S) (C)
1 drop Lavender
1 drop Marjoram
2 drops Chamomile Roman
1 drop Frankincense
5 ml Base oil or cream

Migraines: (V) (I) (C)
1 drop Lavender
1 drop Chamomile Roman
3 drops Marjoram

Haircare

Dandruff: (H)
3 drops Tea Tree
1 drop Rosemary
1 drop Lavender
5 ml Base oil

Thinning hair: (H)
2 drops Lemon
2 drops Clary Sage
1 drop Chamomile Roman
5 ml Jojoba
Mix the ingredients together and massage gently to the scalp (increasing blood flow to the scalp). Leave on the head for a minimum of 30 minutes and rinse off. This treatment can be applied once a week. Alternatively, add this combination of oils to your usual shampoo or conditioner.

physical aromatherapy

Head lice: (H)
2 drops Juniperberry
2 drops Bergamot
1 drop Lavender
5 ml Base oil
Combine the ingredients and work through scalp and hair. It may be necessary to double or triple the recipe if hair is long. Use a nit comb to remove as many larvae as possible and then leave the blend on the hair for at least 30 minutes before washing out. Repeat this treatment every other day until the head lice have been eradicated.

Eyes

To apply, douse a cotton wool ball or pad with the liquid and gently place on the closed eye. Leave in position for a minimum of 10 minutes. Re-apply as often as necessary using a fresh cotton pad for each eye each time to prevent cross infection. If you make up a quantity of your desired blend it's a good idea to refrigerate it to add to its soothing qualities.

Styes (Infected eyelash root):
Lavender Floral Water and Witch Hazel in equal measures

Irritation (dry and itchy) of the eyes:
Chamomile Floral Water or Rose Floral Water

Conjunctivitis:
Lavender Floral Water, Chamomile Floral Water and Witch Hazel in equal measures

Bruising of the eye:
Geranium Floral Water, Chamomile Floral Water and Witch Hazel in equal measures

Ears

Middle ear inflammation:
2 drops Chamomile Roman
2 drops Lavender
1 drop Eucalyptus
5 ml Base oil of choice
Mix together and apply around outer of ear and surrounding area. Dip a little cotton wool into blend and use as an ear plug.

Middle ear infection:
2 drops Tea Tree
2 drops Lavender
1 drop Eucalyptus
5 ml Base oil of choice
Mix together and trickle into the ear, plug with cotton wool. Do not use this method if a perforated ear drum has been diagnosed. If so, apply externally around the whole ear.

Excessive ear wax:
10ml Grapeseed oil
1 drop of Juniperberry
Warm the oil blend very gently to reach blood temperature. Lie on your side and pour the oil into the ear (it's easier if you can get someone to help with this). Stay in position for 10 to 15 minutes and then tip the head to empty the oil from the ear canal. Repeat on opposite ear if needed. After treatment flush the ears gently with warm water – the shower is perfect for this. Any earwax will be broken down to be released naturally of its own accord. Please do not use a cotton bud or anything else to delve into the ear canal as this may impact the wax further and exacerbate the problem.

Tinnitus:
3 drops Juniperberry
1 drop Marjoram
1 drop Chamomile Roman
5 ml Base oil of choice
Mix together and apply around outer of ear and surrounding area. Dip a little cotton wool into blend and use as an ear plug.

Infected ear piercings: (S)
2 drops Tea Tree
2 drops Lavender
1 drop Chamomile Roman
5 ml Base oil or cream of choice

Mouth and teeth

Essential oils have been used for oral care for thousands of years. However, due to their potency it is always recommended to seek the advice of a qualified aromatherapist before oral application. Having said that, it is possible to treat ailments that occur on the lips and dental ailments topically through the external cheek and jaw areas. Naturally it is advisable to visit a dentist and hygienist regularly and especially if you experience any dental problems.

Chapped lips: (S)
1 drop Geranium or Rose Geranium
1 drop Lavender
1 drop Chamomile Roman
5 ml Calendula Infused Oil
Blend together and apply sparingly (so as not to accidentally ingest) as and when needed.

Cold sores: (S)
1 drop Bergamot
1 drop Lemon
1 drop Tea Tree
2 drops Geranium or Rose Geranium
5 ml Base oil of choice
Mix together and apply frequently onto the cold sore with a cotton wool bud (using a fresh bud each time). It is possible to use your finger tip to apply the blend though to prevent further outbreaks or contamination. Wash your hands thoroughly, preferably with a soap containing Tea Tree Oil.

Toothache and abscesses: (S)
1 drop of Clove
1 drop Lavender
3 drops Chamomile Roman
5 ml Base oil or cream
This recipe is ideally for use at onset of any dental pain though dental treatment should be sought as soon as possible. In the case of abscesses a salt water mouth rinse may help to alleviate the pain. Continue to use the blend after treatment to aid healing.

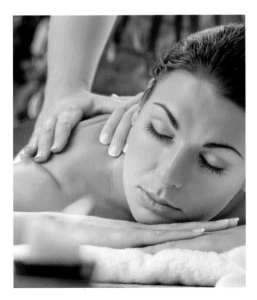

physical aromatherapy

Nose and sinuses

Blocked nose: (I) (T)
Eucalyptus
Ginger
Cedarwood Atlas
Tea Tree

Sinusitis: (S) (I) (T)
1 drop Eucalyptus
1 drop Geranium
1 drop Tea Tree
1 drop Chamomile Roman
1 drop Lavender
5 ml Base oil or cream
Mix together and apply around the
neck, ears, cheekbones, nose and forehead
keeping away from eyes. A blend of
Eucalyptus, Geranium and Tea Tree is
preferable for either the steam inhalation
method or sniffing from a tissue.

Hay fever/allergies: (I) (T)
1 drop Chamomile Roman
1 drop Eucalyptus
1 drop Lemon

Infected nose piercing:
Treat as infected ear piercing.

Neck and throat

**Stiff neck and
shoulder tension: (M) (S) (C)**
2 drops Ginger
1 drop Geranium
1 drop Clary Sage
1 drop Lemongrass
5 ml Base oil or cream

Laryngitis and sore throat: (S) (I) (T)
2 drops Tea Tree
1 drop Eucalyptus
1 drop Lemon
1 drop Lavender
5 ml Base oil or cream
One drop of Sage oil can be substituted
for Eucalyptus in extreme cases but should
never be used on children or pregnant
women.

Digestive system

When treating the abdominal area it is
good practise to apply a topical blend in
the same direction as the digestive tract.
Work in a clockwise motion over the
whole abdomen.

Bloated abdomen: (M)
3 drops Fennel
1 drop Peppermint
1 drop Ginger
5 ml Base oil or cream

Abdominal pain: (M)
upper area:
3 drops Peppermint
1 drop Marjoram
1 drop Clove
5 ml Base oil or cream

Abdominal pain: (M)
lower area: (M)
3 drops Eucalyptus
1 drop Peppermint
1 drop Geranium
1 drop Ginger
5 ml Base oil or cream

Heartburn: (M)
2 drops Eucalyptus
3 drops Peppermint
5 ml Base oil or cream

Nausea: (M)
1 drop Ginger
2 drops Peppermint
2 drops Fennel
5 ml Base oil or cream

Diarrhoea: (M)
2 drops Chamomile Roman
1 drops Cypress
2 drops Eucalyptus
5 ml Base oil or cream

Constipation: (M)
1 drop Marjoram
2 drops Juniperberry
1 drop Fennel
1 drop Orange
5 ml Base oil or cream

Haemorrhoids: (S)
5 drops Cypress
5 ml Base oil or cream

Respiratory system

Common cold: (S) (I) (T) (B)
2 drops Tea Tree
1 drop Lemon
2 drops Eucalyptus
5 ml Base oil or cream

Coughs: (S) (I) (T) (B)
3 drops Frankincense
1 drop Eucalyptus
1 drop Rosemary
5 ml Base oil or cream

Catarrh: (S) (I) (T) (B)
2 drops Eucalyptus
1 drop Peppermint
2 drops Tea Tree
5 ml Base oil or cream

Chest Infections: (S) (I) (T) (B)
1 drop Marjoram
2 drops Tea Tree1 drop Cypress
1 drop Frankincense
5 ml Base oil or cream

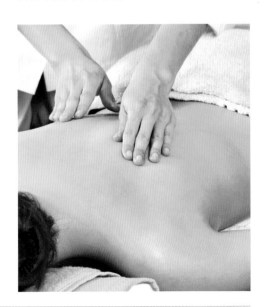

physical aromatherapy

Joint, muscle and back care

Arthritis: (S) (B) (C)
1 drop Juniperberry
2 drops Marjoram
2 drops Chamomile Roman
5 ml Base oil or cream

Bursitis: (S) (B) (C)
2 drops Chamomile Roman
1 drop Cypress
1 drop Ginger
1 drop Juniperberry
5 ml Base oil or cream

Sprains: (S) (C)
1 drop Marjoram
2 drops Lavender
2 drops Chamomile Roman

Back pain: (M) (S) (C)
2 drops Lavender
1 drop Chamomile Roman
1 drop Clary Sage
1 drop Rosemary
5 ml Base oil or cream

Skin

Abrasions and grazes: (S)
1 drop Lavender
1 drop Tea Tree

Follow normal first aid protocol by flushing
the area with plenty of clean water. Swish the
essential oils in more water and dab around
the graze with gauze or cotton wool.

Blisters: (S)
3 drops Lavender
2 drops Chamomile Roman
5 ml Base oil or cream

Boils: (S)
2 drops Bergamot
1 drop Chamomile Roman
2 drops Lavender
5 ml Base oil or cream

Broken veins: (S)
3 drops Chamomile Roman
2 drops Rose Otto
5 ml Base oil or cream

Burns: including sunburn (S)
5 drops Lavender
5 ml Base oil or cream

Nettle rash and stings: (S)
3 drops Lavender
2 drops Chamomile Roman
5 ml Base oil or cream

Eczema dry: (S) (B)
2 drops Lavender
2 drops Chamomile Roman
1 drop Geranium or Rose Geranium
5 ml Base oil or cream

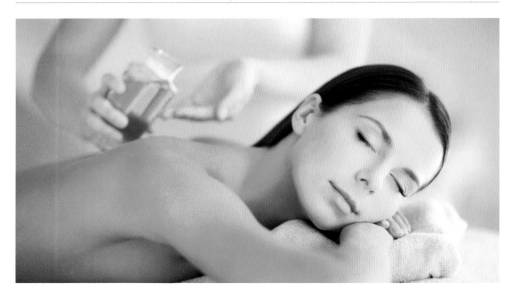

Eczema wet: (S) (B)
2 drops Lavender
2 drops Chamomile Roman
1 drop Juniperberry
5 ml Base oil or cream

Acne: (S)
2 drops Tea Tree
2 drops Lavender
1 drop Juniperberry
5 ml Jojoba Oil

Psoriasis: (S) (B)
3 drops Bergamot
2 drops Chamomile Roman
5 ml Base oil or cream

Insect Bites: (S)
5 drops lavender
5 ml Base oil or cream

Circulation

**Hypertension
(High Blood Pressure) M, S, B, V**
5 drops Marjoram
5 ml Base oil or cream

**Hypotension
(Low Blood Pressure): (M) (S) (B) (V)**
5 drops Sage
5 ml Base oil or cream

Varicose Veins: (S) (B)
3 drops Geranium
2 drops Cypress
5 ml Base oil or cream

Oedema (water retention): (S) (B)
4 drops Juniperberry
1 drop Cypress
5 ml Base oil or cream

Chills: (M) (B)
3 drops Rosemary
2 drops Ginger
5 ml Base oil or cream

physical aromatherapy

Gynaecological

Periods: (S) (B) (V)
Heavy
3 drops Geranium or Rose Geranium
1 drop Lemon
1 drop Chamomile Roman
5 ml Base oil or cream

Scanty
2 drops Clary Sage
2 drops Geranium or Rose Geranium
1 drop Fennel
5 ml Base oil or cream

PMT: (S) (M) (B) (V) (I) (T)
2 drops Clary Sage
2 drops Geranium or Rose Geranium
1 drop Lavender
5 ml Base oil or cream

Menopausal hot flushes:
(S) (M) (B) (V) (I) (T)
2 drops Sage
1 drop Fennel
1 drop Cypress
1 drop Geranium or Rose Geranium
5 ml Base oil or cream

Miscellaneous

Influenza: (S) (M) (B) (V) (I) (T)
2 drops Tea Tree
2 drops Lavender
1 drop Clove
5 ml Base oil or cream

Hangover: (V) (T) (S)
Lemon
Rosemary
Fennel

Overweight: (S) (M) (B) (V) (T)
3 drops Fennel
2 drops Grapefruit
5 ml Base oil or cream

Underweight: (S) (M) (B) (V) (T)
3 drops Lime
2 drops Geranium or Rose Geranium
5 ml Base oil or cream

Fainting: (T)
Rosemary
Lavender

Addiction: (S) (M) (B) (V) (T)
5 drops Bergamot
5 ml Base oil or cream

Cellulite: (S) (M) (B)
3 drops Geranium or Rose Geranium
2 drops Grapefruit
5 ml Base oil or cream

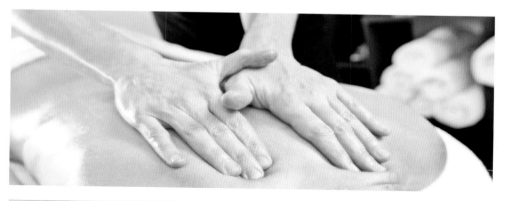

psychological aromatherapy

psychological aromatherapy

Essential oils have been used for centuries to assist with problems of a psychological nature. This at a glance list aims to help you quickly find the best oil to use for a wide range of emotional and psychological issues.

There may be a combination of emotions involved. If so, use those essential oils that are indicated next to all the emotions relevant to you or your patient or create your own blend from those listed.

It's always good practice to sniff test oils before use so you can check that it feels right for you or the person you are treating. Everybody reacts differently to each essential oil so it's worth taking the time to ensure that you have chosen the right oil for the requirements of yourself or the person you are helping.

The oils listed to each condition can be used in massage, vaporised or burned, as a steam inhalation or simply added to a warm bath. For more information on the different techniques for utilising essential oils please see the 'How to use essential oils' chapter.

Absent-mindedness: Lemon, Lime, Cedarwood Atlas to focus and ground.

Acrimony: Lavender, Ylang Ylang to soften the heart.

Aloofness: Frankincense, Geranium or Rose Geranium to enhance trust of oneself and others.

Angst: Bergamot, Lavender, Grapefruit to lift emotions into joyful peace.

Assertion of Emotions: Ginger, Rosemary, Frankincense to increase self-belief.

Assurance: Juniperberry, Lavender, Jasmin to help build confidence.

Bewilderment: Lemon, Patchouli to cut through confusion and ground emotions.

Bravery: Sage, Cedarwood Atlas, Frankincense to strengthen and reassure.

Cabin Fever: Clary Sage, Frankincense, Lemongrass to expand emotional horizons.

Centring: Chamomile Roman, Rose Geranium or Geranium, Frankincense to calm, balance and centre.

Certainty: Rosemary, Grapefruit to clarify decision making.

Confidence: Bergamot, Frankincense to enhance self-belief.

Confusion: Clary Sage, Rosemary to lift emotions out of foggy thinking.

Clear Thinking: Eucalyptus, Grapefruit, Rosemary to sharpen the mind.

Dejection: Lemon, Bergamot, Orange to remind oneself of your own joy.

Delirium: Lavender, Clary Sage, Neroli to calm and cushion emotions in times of immense confusion.

Delusional: Frankincense, Lavender to ground and calm with loving honesty.

Dependency: Cypress, Rose Geranium or Geranium to loosen grip on unhelpful attachments.

psychological aromatherapy

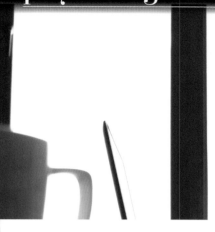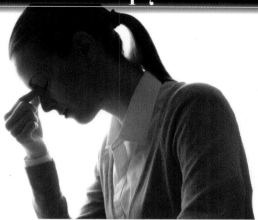

Disappointment: Bergamot, Frankincense, Rose to comfort and lift the heart.

Disinterest: Lemongrass to enliven creative thinking.

Disparaging of the Self: Frankincense, Ylang Ylang, Jasmin to improve low self esteem.

Distrust: Chamomile Roman, Clove to calm and warm emotions towards others.

Enduring Difficulties: Frankincense, Rose to heal heartache and remain trusting.

Enlivened Thinking: Rosemary, Peppermint, Eucalyptus to invigorate the senses.

Equanimity: Frankincense, Patchouli, Rose Geranium or Geranium to centre and balance.

Estrangement: Marjoram, Clary Sage, Frankincense to bring down self-imposed barriers to others.

Explosive Emotions: Chamomile Roman, Neroli to enhance serenity.

Fear of Defeat: Lavender, Cedarwood Atlas to calm and reconnect with self-belief.

Fear of the Future: Rosemary, Jasmin to promote courage.

Fixation: Frankincense to loosen unhealthy over thinking.

Fretting About Past Events: Frankincense, Rose, Lemon to comfort and move emotions forward.

Furtiveness: Ylang Ylang, Grapefruit, Jasmin to open up emotions softly yet fearlessly.

Hastiness: Lavender, Roman Chamomile, Marjoram to slow down into the rhythm of peace.

Heartache: Rose, Neroli, Ylang Ylang to accept with love and release with love.

Hesitancy: Rosemary, Bergamot, Cypress to move forward with positivity.

Hyperactivity: Clary Sage, Marjoram, Lavender to enhance calm and relaxed thinking.

Illogical Thoughts: Lavender, Marjoram, Juniperberry to clear, calm and centre thoughts.

Immediate Calm: Neroli, Frankincense, Lavender to relax instantaneously.

psychological aromatherapy

Incoherence: Ylang Ylang, Lavender to appease irrational emotions.

Inconsistent: Cedarwood Atlas, Frankincense to ground and focus motivations.

Indifference: Clary Sage, Orange, Rosemary to bring joyful focus in discovering another way.

Inflexible Thinking: Orange, Ylang Ylang, Frankincense to encourage open mindedness.

Isolation: Frankincense, Bergamot, Rose to relieve feelings of separation.

Jealousy: Patchouli, Jasmin, Clary Sage to release negativity and remind oneself of one's own unique value.

Lack of Focus: Rosemary, Grapefruit, Sage to clear fogginess and sharpen intention.

Laziness: Rosemary, Juniperberry, Peppermint to lighten emotions and increase purpose.

Lethargy: Rosemary, Lemon, Cypress to invigorate and revive thoughts.

Melancholy: Bergamot, Clary Sage, Rose Geranium or Geranium to increase cheerfulness.

Mental Fatigue: Rosemary, Eucalyptus, Peppermint to maintain focused thinking.

Mood Swings: Lavender, Clary Sage, Rose Geranium or Geranium to stabilise and balance emotions.

Mourning: Rose, Cypress, Neroli to lovingly honour and release grief.

Negative Thinking: Bergamot, Lavender, Orange to promote positive, happy feelings.

Nervous Exhaustion: Patchouli, Clary Sage, Lemongrass to calm and reassure frayed emotions.

Nightmares: Frankincense, Chamomile Roman, Lavender to instil peace to the subconscious mind.

Over Chatty: Cypress, Chamomile Roman, Marjoram to bring stillness and contemplation.

Over Examining: Frankincense, Clary Sage, Lavender to enhance acceptance.

Panic Attacks: Neroli, Lavender, Frankincense to encourage peaceful and tranquil thoughts.

Perceptibility: Grapefruit, Chamomile Roman to enhance intuition.

Performance Anxiety: Lavender, Ylang Ylang, Orange to bring cheerful confidence.

Procrastination: Rosemary, Lemon, Frankincense to continue with courage.

Recklessness: Clary Sage, Frankincense, Rose Geranium or Geranium to keep grounded when overexcited.

Recollection: Rosemary, Grapefruit to enhance memory particularly for study.

Recurring Dreams: Clary Sage, Lavender, Neroli to allow the subconscious mind to let go.

Relaxation: Lavender, Marjoram, Clary Sage to promote deep calm.

Remorse: Rose to reconcile emotions and lovingly forgive.

Renewing: Frankincense, Lemongrass to move forward emotionally.

Rivalry: Orange, Ylang Ylang, Neroli to centre and lighten oneself in self worth.

psychological aromatherapy

Ruefulness: Rose, Bergamot to forgive oneself and move forward.

Safety: Rose, Lavender, Frankincense to enhance feeling of security.

Seductive: Ylang Ylang, Jasmin, Cinnamon (skin caution) to act as aphrodisiacs.

Self-Abasement: Rose Geranium or Geranium, Bergamot, Chamomile Roman to help value oneself.

Self-Approval: Bergamot, Ginger (skin caution), Frankincense to enhance self acceptance.

Self-Doubt: Frankincense, Lavender, Jasmin to improve courage.

Self-Importance: Orange, Lime, Ylang Ylang to increase kindness to others.

Self-Recognition: Rose, Frankincense, Bergamot to connect and accept all of your emotions.

Self-Worth: Cedarwood Atlas, Rose, Ylang Ylang to improve low self esteem.

Scrutiny: Rosemary, Juniperberry, Eucalyptus to enhance concentration.

Shame: Rose, Ylang Ylang, Orange to forgive and release guilt.

Shock: Neroli, Lavender, Marjoram to bring instant tranquillity.

Shielding: Frankincense, Juniperberry, Sage to protect and clear negative energies.

Sleeplessness: Chamomile Roman, Marjoram, Lavender to promote sound sleep.

Sourness: Grapefruit, Orange, Lime to help bring about a sunny outlook.

Stubbornness: Rose Geranium or Geranium, Patchouli, Orange to encourage a balanced yet open attitude.

Sullen: Lemongrass, Bergamot, Clary Sage to uplift emotions and lessen moodiness.

Suspicion of People: Ylang Ylang, Orange, Jasmin to promote trust in others.

Tension: Lavender, Clary Sage, Cedarwood Atlas to bring grounded peacefulness.

Terror: Neroli, Frankincense, Marjoram to lessen fears.

Timidity: Lemon, Jasmin, Fennel to build confidence and open up emotionally.

Tranquillity: Lavender, Chamomile Roman, Neroli to enhance feeling of serenity.

Trepidation: Patchouli, Frankincense, Clary Sage to calm uncertainties and enhance trust.

Unbalanced Emotions: Rose Geranium or Geranium, Lavender, Rose to settle emotions into peace.

Worry: Lavender, Frankincense, Chamomile Roman to calm and centre.

disclaimer

This book is aimed at giving people who have little or no experience in using essential oils the chance to discover and safely use them at home. It is not intended as a definitive reference book, more as a guide to help you start using the oils and other products safely and with confidence.

It's important to remember that while essential oils are safe when properly used, care should always be taken. Because essential oils are absorbed easily into the body it is vital that you ensure that you are not using too much of the oils too often. Most oils are entirely safe, but some require caution as they can build up in the body over time. This is especially true when it comes to making your own blends for application to the skin although essential oils also enter the body via inhalation when burned or vaporised. It is possible to have too much of a good thing!

It is the responsibility of the reader to ensure that the relevant safety protocols have been followed (for example, skin patch testing and the avoidance of using too much of any particular oil too often).

With a safe and cautious approach aromatherapy and essential oils can have an extremely positive effect on the body and mind. But, in the same

way as you wouldn't take more painkiller tablets than stated on the packet, you should ensure that you pay attention to the dilution rate table in this book, that the oil(s) you are using are suitable for the intended application and the person you are treating and keep an eye out for any issues or health problems arising.

Essential oils can be hazardous when taken internally. We would advise that essential oils are never swallowed unless under the express instruction of a qualified aromatherapist. We would also urge caution when using essential oils while pregnant (some oils are safe to use while pregnant but on balance we would recommend that they are avoided altogether in the first trimester of pregnancy and that you ensure any oil you intend to use in the second and third trimester is absolutely safe to use in this period before application) and that they are not used at all on children under the age of 12 months.

If you or anyone that you practise aromatherapy on develops any sort of reaction to the oils or blends that you are using then discontinue their use.

stockists

stockists

Useful links & recommended suppliers

Recommended Suppliers:

UK: Amphora Aromatics Ltd.
www.amphora-aromatics.com

U.S.: Enfleurage
www.enfleurage.com

Australia: Springfields
www.springfieldsaroma.com

Canada: Escents Aromatherapy
www.escentsaromatherapy.com/

Local stockists:

aromatherapy in practice

Useful links:

The International Federation of
Professional Aromatherapists:
www.ifparoma.org/

The International Fragrance Association:
www.ifraorg.org/

The British Essential Oils Association:
www.beoa.co.uk/

National Association for
Holistic Aromatherapy:
www.naha.org/

Aromatherapy & Allied Practitioners
Association:
www.aapa.org.uk/Join.html

The International Federation of
Aromatherapists:
www.ifaroma.org/en/home/

Aromatherapy education courses:
www.itecworld.co.uk/

Federation of Holistic Aromatherapists:
www.fht.org.uk/home/

The Cosmetic, Toiletry and Perfume
Association:
www.ctpa.org.uk/

The International Federation of Essential
Oil and Aroma Trades:
www.ifeat.org/

glossary

glossary

Aromatherapy: The use of essential oils and carrier oils to promote both physical and mental well-being.

Adaptogen: Any natural substance that assists the body in adapting to stress.

Analgesic: Any substance that provides relief from physical pain.

Antihistaminic: Promotes relief from allergies caused by sensitivity or intolerance of proteins.

Antidepressant: Relieves depression. Can help with anxiety and a variety of other nervous or stress related disorders.

Anti-inflammatory: Reduces or prevents inflammation of muscles and skin tissue.

Antimicrobial: Kills or inhibits the growth of microorganisms.

Antineuralgic: Lessens nerve pain.

Anti-oxidant: Prevents the oxidation reactions that can cause harmful free-radicals. Particularly pertinent to skincare.

Antiphlogistic: Anti-inflammatory and also counteracts fever.

Antipruritic: Controls and soothes itching and other skin irritations.

Anti-rheumatic: Helps to relieve rheumatism.

Antiseptic: Prevents the instigation or spread of infection, sepsis or putrefaction.

Antispasmodic: Helps to soothe or prevent muscle spasms.

Antiviral: Inhibits or stops the spread of viral infections.

Antitoxic: Acts to counter toxins and / or poisons.

Aperitif: Stimulating to the appetite.

Aphrodisiac: Increases sexual desire and appetite.

Astringent: Drying and protecting for the skin.

Ayurvedic (Ayurveda): The method of traditional medicinal treatments native to the Indian Subcontinent.

Bactericidal: Kills and prevents the spread of bacteria.

Balsamic: Generally soothing and healing.

Carminative: Prevents build-up of intestinal wind and encourages expulsion of trapped wind.

Cephalic: Stimulates and clears the mind.

Choleretic: Improves the secretion of bile from the liver as well as solids.

Contraindications: Any factor (mainly physiological) that prevents the usage of a certain oil due to an inherent property of the substance which may cause problems with an existing medical condition.

Counterirritant: Creates inflammation in one zone of the body in order to discourage inflammation in another area.

Cuticle (hair): The outermost part of the hair shaft.

Cuticle (nails - eponychium): The thickened layer of skin around the finger and toe nails.

Deodorant: Combats and disguises or removes nasty smells produced by sweat or fungal infections.

Depurative: A purifying and detoxifying action.

Detoxifying: Promotes the removal of toxic substances from a living organism

Diuretic: Encourages and increases the expulsion of urine.

glossary

Emmenagogue: Increases blood flow in the pelvic area and uterus. Some stimulate menstruation and a minority can trigger abortion.

Emollient: Softening to the skin and provides greater elasticity as hydration is improved and helps to replenish the skins natural oils.

Euphoric: Promotes a feeling of happiness and well-being.

Expectorant: Encourages the body to increase the fluidity of substances expelled from the body (specifically the lungs) thus making it easier to clear stubborn mucous as well as soothing the respiratory tract.

Febrifuge: Helps to reduce or prevent fever and high temperature.

Fungicidal: Kills or controls fungal infections.

Galactagogue: Promotes lactation.

Haemostatic: Inhibits bleeding.

Hepatic: Cleansing and detoxifying to the liver.

Hypotensive: Lowers the blood pressure.

Immuno-stimulant: Stimulates the components which activate the immune system

Insecticide: Repels and kills insects.

Insomnia: The inability to get to sleep or to stay asleep for long enough.

Laxative: Promotes the passage of faeces through the bowels. Misuse can cause diarrhoea.

Nervine: Stimulating and strengthening to the nervous system.

Palpitations: Rapid and uncomfortable beating of the heart, sometimes caused by stress both physical and mental.

Parasitic: Assists in the removal of parasites (normally intestinal) from the body.

Prophylactic: Prevents an illness or other medical issue rather than treating or curing it once established.

Restorative: Restores and renews general health and strength.

Rubefacient: Causes dilation of the capillaries and increases blood circulation.

Sebum: The oily, waxy substance produced by the skin that helps to keep skin supple. Overproduction of sebum can lead to greasy skin and / or hair.

Sedative: Calms and reduces irritability and overexcitement.

Sensitisation: The result of over exposure to any substance to which the body is allergic or intolerant.

Stimulant: Promotes improvement (mostly temporary) of both mental and physical processes.

Stomachic: Improves the workings of the stomach and helps to increase appetite.

Sudorific: Promotes and induces sweating.

Tonic: Promotes general health and wellbeing.

Vasoconstrictive: Narrows blood vessels due to contraction of the muscular wall.

Vasodilatory: Relaxes the muscles in the wall of blood vessels and decreases blood pressure while increasing blood flow.

Vermifuge: Encourages the removal of parasitic worms by stunning them.

Vulnerary: Promotes and quickens the healing of wounds.

bibliography

Worwood, Valerie Ann; **The Fragrant Pharmacy,** Bantam Books, London, 1990

Westwood, Christine; **Aromatherapy – A Guide for Home Use**, Amberwood, Guildford, 1991

Davids, Patricia; **Aromatherapy – An A-Z,** Vermilion, London, 1988

Lawless, Julia; **The Encyclopedia of Essential Oils**, Element, Shaftesbury, 1992

Tucker, Louise; **An Introductory Guide to Aromatherapy,** London, 2000

Higley, Connie & Alan, Leatham, Pat; **Aromatherapy A-Z**, Hay House, 1998

Borseth, Kolbjørn; **The Aromantic Guide to unlocking the powerful health & rejuvenation benefits of vegetable oils,** Aromantic Ltd, 2008

Liz Earle; **Vital Oils,** Vermillion, 1992

Westwood, Christine; **Aromatherapy Stress Management**, Amberwood, 1993

notes

notes

notes

notes

notes

notes

aromatherapy in practice

index

A

Abdominal 138
Abrasions 139
Absent-mindedness 144
Absolute 107
Absolutes 22
Acne 140
Acrimony 144
Adaptogen 150
Addiction 141
Allergies 137
Aloofness 144
Amyris balsamifera 98
Analgesic 150
Angst 144
Anthemis nobilis 44
Antidepressant 150
Antihistaminic 150
Anti-inflammatory 150
Antimicrobial 150
Antineuralgic 150
Anti-oxidant 150
Antiphlogistic 150
Antipruritic 150
Anti-rheumatic 150
Antiseptic 150
Antispasmodic 150
Antitoxic 150
Antiviral 150
Aperitif 150
Aphrodisiac 150
Argan 120
Argania spinosa 120
Aromatherapy: 150
Arthritis 139
Assertion of Emotions 144
Assurance 144
Astringent 150
Avicenna 22
Avocado 120
Ayurveda 150
Ayurvedic 150

B

Back 139
Back pain 139
Bactericidal 150
Balsamic 150
Base product 36
Bergamot 40
Bewilderment 144
Blisters 139
Bloated abdomen 137
Blocked nose 137
Boils 139
Boswellia carterii 62
Bravery 144
Broken veins 139
Bruising of the eye 135
Burns 139
Bursitis 139
Buxus chinensis 123

C

Cabin Fever 144
Calendula 108
Calendula officinalis 108
Cananga odorata 104
Carminative 150
Carrier oils 120
Catarrh 138
Cedarwood atlas 42
Cedrus atlantica 42
Cellulite 141
Centring 144
Cephalic 150
Certainty 144
Chamomile. *See* Ch
Chamomile roman 44
Chapped lips 136
Chest Infections 138
Chills 140
Choleretic 150
Cinnamomum zeylanicum 46
Cinnamon 46

index

Circulation 140
Citronella 48
Citrus aurantifolia 80
Citrus Aurantium 112
Citrus aurantium dulcis 86
Citrus bergamia 40
Citrus limon 76
Citrus nobilis 82
Citrus paradisi 68
Clary sage 50
Clear Thinking 144
Clove 52
Cold sores 136
Common cold: 138
Confidence 144
Confusion 144
Conjunctivitis 135
Constipation 138
Contraindications 150
Coughs 138
Counterirritant 150
Cupressus Sempervirens 54
Cuticle 150
Cymbopogon Winterianus 48
Cypress 54

D

Dejection 144
Delirium 144
Delusional 144
Deodorant 150
Dependency 144
Depurative 150
Detoxifying 150
Diarrhoea 138
Digestive 137
Dilution 36
Disappointment 145
Disinterest 145
Disparaging of the Self 145
Distrust 145
Diuretic 150

E

Ears 135
Eczema dry 139
Eczema wet 140
Emmenagogue 151
Emollient 151
Emotions 144
Enduring Difficulties 145
Enlivened Thinking 145
Eponychium 150
Equanimity 145
Estrangement 145
Eucalyptus 56
Eucalyptus globulus 56
Eugenia caryophyllus 52
Euphoric 151
Evening primrose 122
Excessive ear wax 135
Expectorant 151
Explosive Emotions 145
Eyes 135

F

Fainting 141
Fear of Defeat 145
Fear of the Future 145
Febrifuge 151
Fennel 60
Fixation 145
Floral waters 128
Foeniculum vulgare 60
Folding 24
Frankincense 62
Fretting About Past Events 145
Fungicidal 151
Furtiveness 145

G

Galactagogue 151
Gamma linoleic acid 122
Geranium 64, 130
Ginger 66

Grapefruit 68
Grapeseed 122
Grazes 139
Gynaecological 141

H

Haemorrhoids 138
Haemostatic 151
Haircare 134
Hangover 141
Hastiness 145
Hay fever 137
Headaches 134
Head lice 135
Heartache 145
Heartburn 138
Heavy 141
Hepatic 151
Hesitancy 145
High Blood Pressure 140
Hot 141
Hydrocarbon 22
Hydrolate 22
Hydrolates 128
Hydrosols 128
Hyperactivity 145
Hypertension 140
Hypotension 140
Hypotensive 151

I

Illogical Thoughts 145
Immediate Calm 145
Immuno-stimulant 151
Incoherence 146
Inconsistent 146
Indifference 146
Infected 137
Infected ear 136
Infected ear piercings 136
Inflexible Thinking 146
Influenza 141
Insect Bites 140

Insecticide 151
Insomnia 151
Irritation 135
Isolation 146

J

Jasmin 110, 130
Jasminum officinale 110
Jealousy 146
Joint 139
Jojoba 123
Juniperberry 70
Juniperus communis 70

K

Kaolin 128

L

Lack of Focus: 146
Laryngitis 137
Lavender 72
Lavendula Angustifolia 72
Laxative 151
Laziness 146
Lemon 76
Lethargy 146
Lime 80
Low Blood Pressure 140
M
Mandarin 82
Marjoram 84
Melalueca alternifolia 100
Melancholy 146
Menopausal 141
Mental Fatigue 146
Mentha arvensis 90
Middle ear infection 135
Middle ear inflammation 135
Migraines 134
Miscellaneous 141
Mood Swings 146
Mourning 146
Mouth and teeth 136

index

Muscle 139

N

Nausea 138
Neck 137
Negative Thinking 146
Neroli 112, 130
Nervine 151
Nervous Exhaustion 146
Nettle rash 139
Nightmares 146
Nose 137

O

Oedema 140
Oenethera biennis 122
Orange 86
Origanum majorana 84
Over Chatty 146
Over Examining 146
Overweight 141

P

Palpitations 151
Panic Attacks 146
Parasitic 151
Patchouli 88
Pelargonium graveolens 64, 92
Peppermint 90
Perceptibility 146
Performance Anxiety 146
Periods 141
Persea gratissima 120
Persistent headaches 134
Physical 134
Piercing 137
PMT 141
Pogostemon cablin 88
Precious 107
Procrastination 146
Prophylactic 151
Prunus amygdalus dulcis 124
Psoriasis 140

Psychological 144

R

Recklessness 146
Recollection 146
Recurring Dreams 146
Relaxation 146
Remorse 146
Renewing 146
Restorative 151
Rivalry 146
Rosa Canina 123
Rosa centifolia 114
Rosa damascena 116
Rosamarinus officinalis 94
Rose 130
Rose geranium 92
Rosehip 123
Rose maroc 114
Rosemary 94
Rose otto 116
Rubefacient 151
Ruefulness 147

S

Safety 147
Sage 96
Salvia officinalis 96
Salvia sclarea 50
Sandalwood Amyris 98
Scanty 141
Scrutiny 147
Sebum 151
Sedative 151
Seductive 147
Self-Abasement 147
Self-Approval 147
Self-Doubt 147
Self-Importance 147
Self-Recognition 147
Self-Worth 147
Sensitisation 151
Shame 147

Shielding 147
Shock 147
Shoulder tension 137
Sinuses 137
Sinusitis 137
Sleeplessness 147
Sore throat 137
Sourness 147
Sprains 139
Steam Distillation 22
Stiff neck 137
Stimulant 151
Stings 139
Stomachic 151
Stress related headaches 134
Stubbornness 147
Styes 135
Sudorific 151
Sullen 147
Sunburn 139
Suspicion of People 147
Sweet almond 124

T

Tea tree 100
Tension 147
Terror 147
Thinning hair 134
Throat 137
Timidity 147
Tinnitus 136
Toner 128
Tonic 151
Toothache and abscesses 136
Tranquillity 147
Trepidation 147
Triticum vulgare 124

U

Unbalanced Emotions 147
Underweight 141

V

Varicose Veins 140
Vasoconstrictive 151
Vasodilatory 151
Vermifuge 151
Vitis vinifera 122
Vulnerary 151

W

Worry 147

Y

Ylang ylang 104

Z

Zingiber officinale 66